LEARNING
HOW
TO
BREATHE

by

DR. CORINNE E. WEAVER, DC

Unless otherwise indicated, all Scripture quotations marked NIV are taken from the Holy Bible, New International Version.

LEARNING HOW TO BREATHE

ISBN:1539705192

ISBN-13: 978-1539705192

Dr. Corinne E. Weaver, DC

14015-D East Independence Blvd.

Indian Trail, NC 28079

Websites: www.drcorinneweaver.com

www.getwellnc.com

DISCLAIMER

The educational information and guidelines contained in this book are based upon the research and the personal and professional experiences of the author. They are not intended as a substitute for consultation with your health care provider. This information is for educational purposes only, and has not been evaluated by the Food and Drug Administration. These products and information are not intended to diagnose, treat, cure, or prevent disease.

DEDICATION

I dedicate this book to my wonderful husband and our three children. Thanks for allowing me to fulfill my dreams and enjoy the benefits of healthy living. Thanks to my kids. Noah, who made me strive harder to live life without the need of drugs. My two amazing daughters; Cora and Sara, who help me stay on my toes with creativity. I am blessed to say they have no need for drugs (medication) in their lives, and I hope to keep it that way. To my mom, Vivian, whose smile and laughter lit up the world. She loved the movie, *The Wizard of Oz*, and I keep reminding my kids there is no place like home. I know my mom is somewhere over the rainbow, and I will see her again soon.

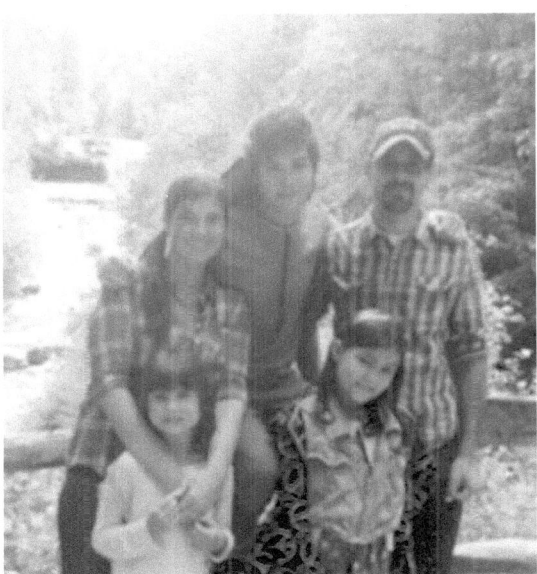

ENDORSEMENTS

Congratulations to Dr. Corinne Weaver, who was recently named one of Charlotte's top doctors for 2016, as seen in the Charlotte magazine. It all started as a youngster when she always strived to do her best, following the example set by her father Don, and of course her uncle John who had an influence in the direction of her future. Her Uncle John had a great desire to help people and became an entrepreneur by starting his own business which grew to be a world renowned leader in his field and he became known as Amazon John. Dr. Weaver's greatest discovery was when she found Jesus Christ and accepted Him as her personal savior; her faith in God has pointed the way for her to help others. With the help and encouragement of her husband, Scott, she graduated from college "Cum Laude" with the degree of Dr. Corinne Weaver, DC as a chiropractor. She too, started her own business, guiding it thru hardships, up and downs, but never becoming discouraged, and letting each hardship lead to a greater success and after many years of cutting-edge technological care is now the author of this book, *Learning How to Breathe*.

So you thought that you already knew how to breathe? As a approach my ninety-three birthday I have learned so much from her and you will too by reading the content of this book. I am proud and very much honored to call Dr. Weaver my granddaughter.

Tom Easterling
Author of "Furrow in the Clouds"

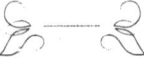

Breathing, you'll never take it for granted again!

Dr. Weaver fills the pages with personal stories and practical tips to reverse disease processes and maximize your life all starting with breath.

'Amazon John' Easterling

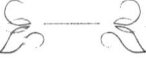

Dr. Corinne Weaver early on acknowledges from scriptures, Is. 26:8, her passion--knowing Jesus and making Him known or renown as key to her successful and rewarding lifestyle and business-ministry. Dr. Weaver shares her personal Jesus story (Rev. 19:10c) of her encounters with Him, how He took her terrible childhood accident and its residual effects and changed her life forever, a Rom. 8:28 experience. He gave her an overwhelming passion to use her experiences and "healing hands" to change others' lives. *Learning How to Breathe* is a practical account from her life experiences, her life's lessons, and testimonials from clients that give hope and life changing tried and practical solutions for *Learning How to Breathe* which is a major key to life, itself. It's a story of listening to God and acting on His promise. Dr. Weaver's passion for Jesus, her family, for life, and helping others help themselves permeates the book—it's indeed epic.

Gerald S. Broome, Sr.,
President and Pastor, Quest Ministries, Monroe, NC 28110

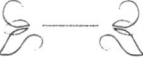

Great Job Dr. Weaver!! Vital information for your highest potential health and a great read! All of the mystery has been taken out of the art of breathing. Your personal story makes it easy to relate and I loved all the extra health tips.

Dr. Robert Kessinger, DC, DABCI, DACBN

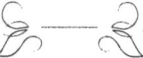

As a mom and a doctor, Dr. Corinne Weaver has a special love for children and to see all children grow up healthy. Her passion, her heart, and her knowledge come through powerfully in the pages of this book. Regardless of your knowledge level, *Learning How to Breathe* provides a wealth of information both for the person wanting to start a healthy lifestyle and for the established health professional.

This is especially a must-read for parents who desire to start their family on a life free of drugs and full of health.

Dr. Weaver's life journey makes her uniquely qualified to offer insight and expert advice in the ways of natural health.

Dr. Michael Anderson, DC

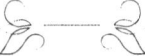

Hold on to your breath and grasp life changing strategies that Dr. Corinne Weaver e.aborately outlines in *Leaning How to Breathe*. I have known her fcr well over eighteen years and I am very blessed to call her a friend and fellow leader in healthcare. Dr. Weaver has eloquently breathed the words into this book so you as the reader can put these health giving principles into action. The ideas set forth in her series of books will lead readers with increased knowledge towards better health and a more enjoyable quality of life. I highly recommenc this book and her many books to come!

Dr. Stephen A. Conicello DC, PSc.D
Functional Medicine
Functional Neurology

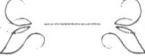

Refreshing to see and hear the basic concepts of health portrayed in a way so easily understood, Great Job Dr. Corinne.

Dr. Greg Melvin, DC
Board Certified Clinical Thermologist

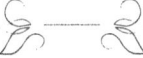

I want to encourage everyone to read this inspiring book, for I believe it can help you throughout your life's journey.

Thank you Dr. Weaver for sharing your healing stories and being a true gift to healthcare.

Olivia Newton-John, OBE, AO

ACKNOWLEDGMENTS

I want to thank first my husband, Scott, who has stood by my side every step of our journey. His constant encouragement has made me realize I can do all things through Christ, who strengthens me. He helps bring balance to my life in our imperfect world.

Thanks Dad, for always telling me to go after my dreams and believing in me. Your support over the years means so much.

Thanks to my grandfather, who also wrote a book, called *Furrow in the Clouds*. He shared his story of being a fighter pilot in WWII and a prisoner of war. Without his fight for survival, I would not be here. I am so honored to be his granddaughter.

I want to thank my Uncle John who inspired me to learn about natural healing. That path led me to a healthier yellow brick road to the Emerald City but once a got there I realized I had all the power inside myself to heal just like Dorothy.

On your pathway to wellness, remember to enjoy the journey. You never know who you might meet along the way. Lions and tigers and bears...oh my!!

Dr. Corinne E. Weaver, DC
October 2016

TABLE OF CONTENTS

PREFACE

I'm 10 years old riding my brand-new pink bicycle. All of a sudden, a horsefly lands on my shoulder. I reach over to knock the horsefly off my shoulder and boom. Next thing I know, I'm flying over my handlebars. I wake up and realize I'm in a hospital, my front tooth is gone, and I can't breathe. That day changed my life forever. I've dedicated all my years since to the study of breathing, helping more than 120,000 patients breathe better. I was living on breathing machines twice a day, with an inhaler in my pocket at my wake and call. That was my life. I then became allergic to everything. My parents had to get rid of our cats, carpet, stuffed animals, and lots more. We had to stop going to our old church because it was moldy, and I had an asthma attack every time we went. My grandmother had to remove all of her flowers and potpourri when we came over. I was always living on the edge not knowing when I would have another attack. It was so scary being a kid struggling to breathe. I thought there was no end.

My amazing Uncle John from the Amazon Jungle would come to town and make me some fresh herbal tea. I breathed in the vapor from that tea with a kitchen towel over my head, and my lungs would open up and alleviate my most severe breathing symptoms. I knew as a small kid I liked breathing in that tea better than the nasty steroid breathing machine I used. Even though the taste of the roots and barks were disgusting, I would take them in, because after I did, I felt better. I knew something was powerful within those herbs he gave me. Even as a small child, I knew I wanted to be a doctor. I thought at one point I would be a pediatrician because I loved children. But as a sick child I **hated** to go see my pediatrician because I didn't like the way the drugs made me feel. I later learned that these drugs increased my heart rate, blood pressure, headaches, blurred vision; exacerbate diabetes, glaucoma, obesity, liver damage, and heart disease.

John gave me the first hope that I could get off these breathing machines, inhalers, and allergic shots. As the years went by, my asthma and allergies got worse with all the added drugs and shots I was on, and I started passing out and having seizures. While visiting my uncle one summer, everything became clear. He had fractured his back in a car accident. As he was lying on the couch in pain, I felt the need to help him. I used recovery herbs on his back and worked on aligning his energy in his spine. He woke up and felt the best he had felt since the accident. He looked at me and said, "You have healing hands." I felt empowered to help others feel better with my hands. He introduced me to chiropractic. I feel in love with the philosophy of chiropractic!! Our bodies have the power to heal from the inside. The power that made the body can heal the body. The nervous system runs the whole body, and if there is no interference with the brain to body communication, the body can operate at its optimum.

As I aged, I developed a strong relationship with God. I prayed at a summer Christian camp called Camp Quest, "Lord what do you want me to be when I grow up?" I heard the word LOUD and CLEAR in my mind – CHIROPRACTOR!

LISTEN: Part of our job is to listen well to the Word of God and the Spirit of God. We are good at talking to God but not listening to God. From that day, on I dedicated my life to help others with their healing.

God promises that if we pursue Him, He will not only provide for our needs (Matthew 6:33) but will give us our desires as well (Psalm 37:4-5). I now understand that bike accident or horsefly was not a coincidence. It was my destiny.

I married my high school sweetheart and went to college based on the philosophy of Chiropractic. Chiropractic was founded on the belief system that the brain & body are intelligently designed to coordinate all necessary aspects of health. Think about it: if you get a cut on your hand, your body knows how to fix it; if you eat something spoiled, your body expels the food by vomitting and/or diarrhea (it isn't pleasant, but it is your body's smart decision to get rid of the toxic food).

From this basic premise, the founders deductively reasoned all the other fundamentals of chiropractic philosophy. These have not changed in over 100 years, and still people all over the world continue to experience their true health potential through chiropractic!

While in chiropractic school, I started receiving regular chiropractic care, specifically, upper cervical care. All my asthma/allergy symptoms disappeared within a year, and I threw all my meds away, and have not gone back for over 16 years. I finished school and opened my practice in 2004. I gave birth to three wonderful children, all of them natural at home, and with no **drugs**. I also love helping women have natural childbirths and educating parents on how to raise healthy children naturally.

In 2005, my Mom was diagnosed with brain cancer and was given 3 months to live. My uncle gave her the best herbs possible, and we worked on her spiritually, physically and mentally, every day. She lost her battle to cancer 3 years later instead of 3 months. But WOW, did my life change fast. Here I was, just opening my new practice and moved back from home, and then my mom got cancer.

In 2012, my vision expanded and shifted to my health again because my health was in decline due to me taking care of everyone else. I was 60 pounds overweight and very fatigued.

Once again, my main problems were detected through a series of diagnostic testing, and I was able to turn my life around. It has made me a better doctor to help patients with those areas of concern. Even though my specialty is in upper cervical spine, I explain and educate my patients in all areas of lifestyle, like stress management, nutrition, cooking, detox, herbal-o-logy, and exercise. Being able to work with other doctors in my network has expanded my knowledge on health.

I absolutely love what I do, and am excited to get this great news out to all of you.

Isaiah.... 26:8

Yes, Lord, walking in the way of your laws, we wait for you; your name and renown are the desire of our hearts.

This book is a start, and I pray it speaks to you and you can wake up each morning with a purpose. What I do every day is a calling, and I give God the glory for allowing his gifts to work through me. I do believe in miracles because I get to see them every day!!!!

As my aunt, Olivia Newton-John Easterling would sing "NOT GONNA GIVE IN TO IT" and Sometimes there is a miracle just beyond the pain and you can see the rainbow in the rain....LIVE ON!!!

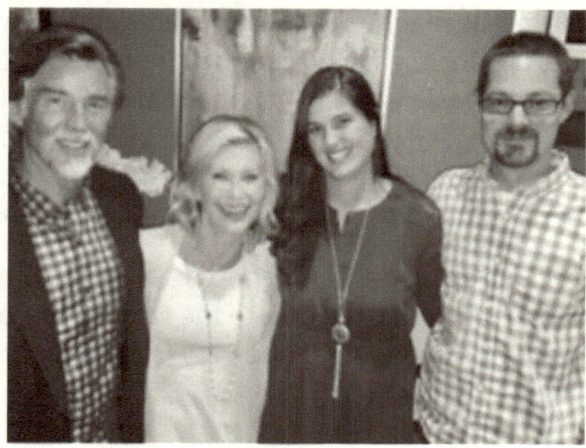

DISCLOSURE ABOUT CASE STUDIES IN THIS BOOK

I have included some case studies in this book from my own practice. These specific case studies were intentionally chosen to help you relate to actual patients and their lives. I shared this book with several of my patients before its release, and they said these stories gave them hope when there was none. We have to have hope when we are improving our health, even though these concepts are not guaranteed to help everyone. I hope these case studies motivate and provide positive energy to assist you on your journey. Follow the yellow brick road…

Chapter 1

ARE YOU MAKING THESE THREE COMMON MISTAKES WHEN YOU BREATHE?

I believe I can trace every ailment we face today to improper breathing. I will be sharing some stories of my patients I have seen over the last 12 years in practice. I hope these stories will speak to your heart and motivate you to take a DEEP BREATH.

According to Men's Journal, "Modern life causes the average person to use about a third of his natural lung capacity."

And the question I want to ask you is: Are you making one of these three common mistakes when you breathe?

1. Time- We are not taking the time to take deep breaths. We're always on the go. I understand. I have three kids and am constantly dropping them here and there. The good thing is, you don't have to take a lot of time to breathe. All you need is a pair of lungs and a few minutes a day. You can train your body to take deep belly breaths throughout the day. The more you take deep breaths, the more natural deep breathing at ease becomes. When we have better control of our breathing, we can lower our blood pressure and help our bodies de-stress. When you are under a lot of stress, it is very hard to control your breath, so practice deep breathing now, and you will have better control when stress comes. Later in the book, I will tell you how you can do these breathing exercises anytime and anyplace.

1

2. Posture. We are always looking down at our cell phones and at our computer screens, causing our posture to be overly flexed forward, which restricts our diaphragm. So many patients I see today wear their shoulders as earrings and are so tight in their upper neck and spine. Later, I will show you what exercises and stretches to do to help you with your posture.

That head trauma from my bicycle accident caused my head to be forward over my shoulders, and not straight. That position caused my lung capacity to drop down by at least 30%.

3. Chemicals. We wake up in the morning and use heavy, artificially-scented shampoos and soaps. We put deodorant with toxic aluminum under our arms that clogs up our lymphatic system. We're using dryer sheets with artificial scents to make our clothes smell. And all these chemicals are closing up our pores and not allowing our body to breathe properly.

Some of the most common recurrent ailments suffered by Americans are allergic reactions to inhaled substances (1). Reactions such as red, itchy eyes; sneezing; and sinus headache are experienced by up to 75 million Americans with seasonal allergies. According to a report published by the American College of Allergy, Asthma, and Immunology (ACAAI), a shortage of physicians specializing in allergies will prevail until nearly 2020 (2).

This will increase the need for more doctors trained in alternative medicine to deal directly with patients needing symptom relief from allergies. In this book, I will show you a number of lifestyle, diet, and non-drug approaches that will help you regain your breath back, and with fewer side effects than conventional allergy medication.

Now that we know these three common mistakes, here is what you should do with your B-R-E-A-T-H...

Dr. Weaver's **B-R-E-A-T-H** System

B-ack

R-elax

E-ssential Oils

A-llergies

T-hermography

H-eal from Inside

Chapter 2

B-ACK

The first letter of my B-R-E-A-T-H system is *B for Back*. You have to have the correct posture in order to breathe properly. There is a nerve in the brainstem called the Vagus. It helps communication from the brain to the body. It controls not only our breathing, but many other life necessities, like our heartbeat.

At the age of 21, I found an upper cervical chiropractor who made adjustment to my upper cervical spine, where the Vagus nerve is located, and for the first time in 11 years, I was able to breathe again without any drugs.

Most people have heard of the "fight or flight" response of the nervous system, the way in which the body reacts to stress or being scared. Many, however, have never heard of the "rest and digest" response. This system, where the Vagus nerve is located, activates the more relaxed functions of the body; those that help maintain a healthy, long-term balance in life.

These systems are both part of a larger system named the autonomic nervous system, which controls and influences the way that our internal organs function. While we all think we have just one nervous system, we actually have several.

If you are suffering from a lot of stress, chances are that your "fight or flight" response has been activated far too often in the past. These kinds of stressors prompt the body to release large amounts of stress hormones, like cortisol. Over the longer term, chronically-elevated stress levels lead to your body organs becoming depleted of the materials that they need to produce key hormones and neurotransmitters for healthy brain function.

The two parts of the Autonomic Nervous System

The sympathetic nervous system, or the "fight or flight" response, prepares our body for these actions. All of the organs involved in getting ready for a physical challenge ("fight") or preparing for a retreat ("flight") are activated through this system. The parasympathetic nervous system ("rest and digest") helps produce a state of equilibrium or balance in the body. Both are part of the greater autonomic nervous system, which is responsible for involuntary and reflexive functions in the body.

The Sympathetic Nervous System

The sympathetic nervous system is faster-acting than the parasympathetic system, and moves along very short, fast neurons. The sympathetic nervous system activates a part of the adrenal gland, which then releases hormones into the bloodstream. These hormones activate the target muscles and glands, causing the body to speed up and become very tense, as well as more alert and ready. Functions that are not immediately essential, like the immune system and digestive system, are shut down to some degree.

Your body goes through a number of changes when the sympathetic nervous system is activated.

- Your heart rate increases
- The bronchial tubes in your lungs dilate
- Your pupils dilate
- Your muscles contract
- Your saliva production is reduced

- Your stomach stops many of the functions of digestion
- More glycogen is converted to glucose

These changes are designed to make you more ready to fight or run from a bear. Non-essential systems, like digestion and immunity, are given much lower priority, while more energy is made available to your muscles, and your heart rate increases. This is what happens when we are faced with a stressor.

The Parasympathetic Nervous System

The parasympathetic, or "rest and digest," system is a much slower system that moves along longer pathways. The parasympathetic response is responsible for controlling homeostasis, or the balance and maintenance of the body's systems. It restores the body to a state of calmness and allows it to relax and repair.

The body undergoes several specific responses when the parasympathetic system is activated.

- Your saliva is increased
- Digestive enzymes are released
- Your heart rate drops
- The bronchial tubes in your lungs constrict
- Your muscles relax
- The pupils in your eyes constrict
- Your urinary output increases

All of these changes are designed to maintain long-term health, improve digestion, conserve energy, and maintain a healthy balance in your body's systems.

How are these systems activated?

The sympathetic nervous system kicks in automatically, and occurs in response to any thought of fear. This doesn't have to be an imminent physical threat (we face those very rarely these days). Any perceived threat or stressful situation can trigger this response. For example, if you have ever felt your heart racing and your mouth dry up ahead of a public speaking engagement, then you know what a sympathetic nervous response feels like. In this example, hormones released by the adrenal glands tell your heart to speed up, and restrict digestive processes like saliva production.

The sympathetic nervous system protects us from real physical dangers like lions, tigers, and bears, oh my, or a threatening scarecrow. However, it can also be triggered by the ordinary stressors we face on a daily basis. These might be things like work or school deadlines, waking up late and missing an activity, or fixing dinner at holiday get-togethers.

Many diseases and illnesses have been shown to stem from chronic stress. Cardiovascular issues, high blood pressure, and immune system suppression are classic symptoms. Other symptoms include constipation and digestive issues, cold sores, jitteriness, sweats, and anxiety. In the longer term, more advanced adrenal fatigue can lead to symptoms like chronically low energy levels, respiratory problems, decreased sexual function, and much more.

The less time we spend in the sympathetic response mode, the better. Although it makes us alert and better able to respond to the challenges ahead, it takes a huge toll on our bodies after a while, and can lead to adrenal burnout and can crash down. Anything we can do to keep ourselves in the "rest and digest" mode as much as possible is worth the effort, since our long-term health may depend on it.

To activate your parasympathetic nervous system, learn what truly makes you feel relaxed. Have fun and engage in a hobby, hang out with friends, exercise, or even just get out into nature and listen to the birds sing. Whatever it is, pay close attention to your feelings and thoughts, and try to recreate those special moments so you can relive them.

We are all under some level of chronic stress these days. By learning to activate your parasympathetic nervous system, and reducing the effect of your sympathetic nervous system, you can reduce the stress on your heart, digestive system, immune system, and more. This will not only make you a happier person, it will also help to avoid many of the diseases and conditions that are associated with chronic stress and adrenal fatigue. If you can become more conscious of the way that your body reacts to stress, it will pay enormous dividends in the future.

We know beyond any doubt stress can be detrimental to our health, and record numbers of us now report feeling stressed. It might be work related, family issues, or simply having a lot on our plates, but stress is something we need to combat if we are to lead healthy, happy lives.

HELPFUL TIPS

Just as we can exercise some control over the sympathetic nervous system (just thinking of a public speaking engagement can trigger a response for many people), we can also activate the parasympathetic nervous system. Simply reading a book does the trick for some people, which may be why so many people read before going to bed for the night. Just pay attention to your posture while you read in bed.

Soaking in a hot bath with Epsom salt and lavender, getting a massage, or petting a dog or cat are good relaxation strategies. I love doing yoga and wall or snow angels daily. See below for these stretches.

Here are some stretches I give to my patients to help them with their posture. If they can't perform these wall angels correctly the first time, I tell them to keep working on it. There are always surprised when they can't do these correctly because they look so easy.

As we age, we get stiffer and should work harder on our flexibility. As someone works on these exercises and stretches, they become taller, and their muscles become more relaxed. When you practice correct posture, your body is in better alignment and can communicate better with the brain. Also, sitting and standing tall can boost up your self-confidence.

Before you start these exercises, visualize a balloon string coming from the top of your head, pulling you gently up towards a ceiling. Visualization is always a good start. No one wants to see themselves as a hunchback or refer to an old granny with a cane. Avoid slouching when sitting and walking at all times.

Start thinking you are a beautiful model. I went to some modeling classes as a kid, and the instructors told us to practice balancing a book on your head. It looked easy, but of course, it was very hard. Having good posture takes time and effort.

My muscles were very tired when I first started these exercises, but over time, it has become part of my daily routine and is easier. My healthiest patients that are in their 80s and 90s do these stretches and exercises every morning. They tell me with a smile how much they love doing them and how it has helped with their flexibility and pain levels.

If you want to change your breathing, it starts with making small, simple commitments each day. I will be going over lots of things I do daily, but I advise you to start small and change one thing at a time. If you change one positive movement in your life now, years of time ahead, you will still put on your shoes by reaching your feet, and move forward in your life to greater wellness.

The key ingredient here is to add something new to your life. It wasn't there before, but you can commit to it, and it will bring more joy in your life in some way.

I have been using the website Fitness Blender for many years now, and I just love it. I have used lots of their exercise programs, and I love that I can do them in the comfort of my home.

Here is one I share with my patients daily. It is called the Better Posture Workout - Exercises to Improve Posture and Prevent Hunched Shoulders.

Here is the link on YouTube.

https://m.youtube.com/watch?v=ahPse5W9Eyo

WALL or SNOW ANGELS

1. Either standing against the wall or lying or your back, bend your knees until your feet are positioned flat on the floor.
2. Pull your shoulders down toward your hips. Try not to arch your back or lift your hips.
3. Bring your arms away from your sides to about 45-degrees, palms rotated toward the ceiling.
4. Gently slide your arms along the wall or floor to an overhead position to a point where your head can touch the wall or floor and your elbows have a comfortable bend.
5. Gently bring your arms back to your starting position, using the same movement pattern.
6. Make sure your elbows and wrists touch the wall or floor. Take a deep breath in and bring your arms up, then exhale while bringing your arms down and squeeze your shoulder blades together. Repeat 10-15 times daily.

WALL ANGELS

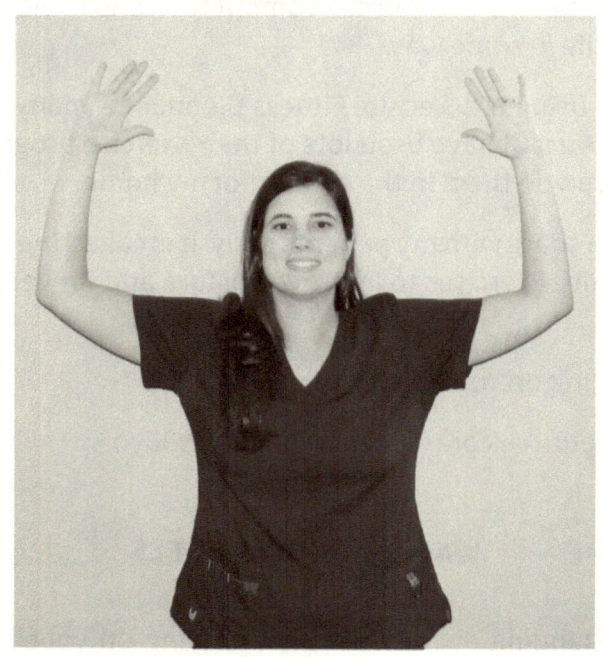

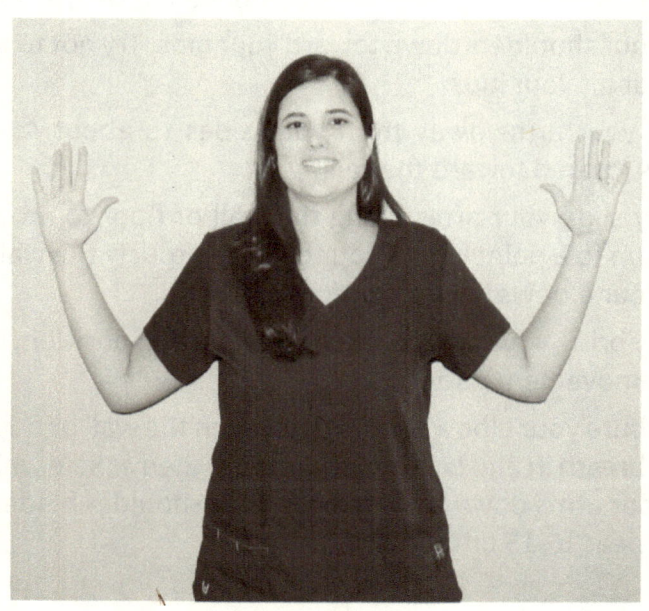

SNOW ANGELS

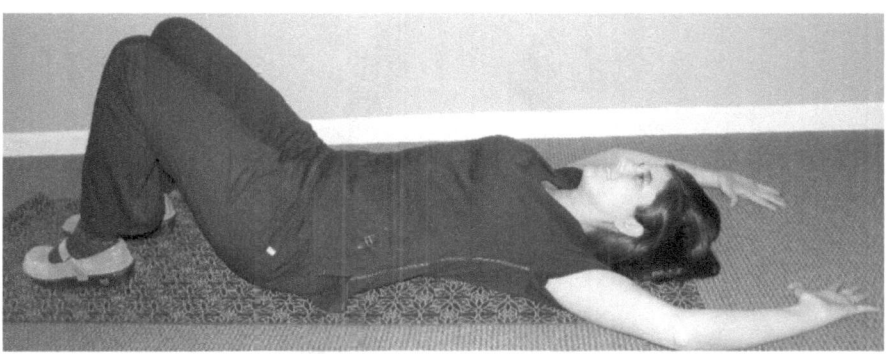

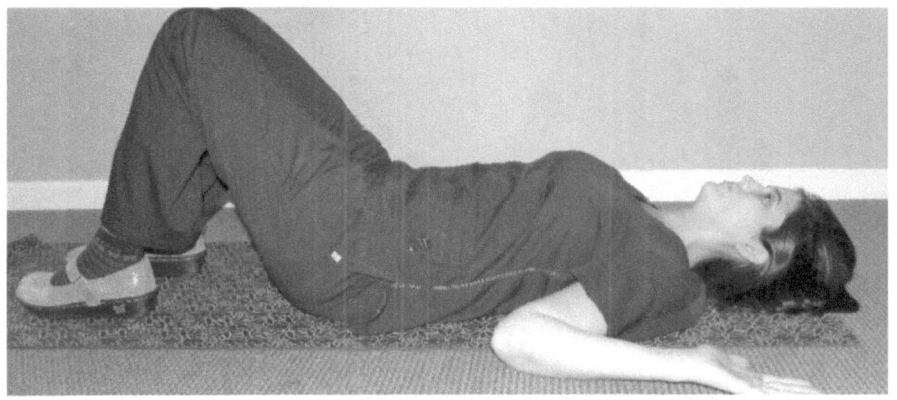

SHOULDER ROLLS

This stretch can be done sitting or standing.

1. Keep your arms hanging loosely at your sides.
2. Raise your shoulders up towards your ears, and then roll them backwards. When rolling your shoulders backwards, try to pinch your shoulder blades together.
3. Hold this position for 2 to 3 seconds.
4. Then relax anc repeat (10 sets (set is a repetitive movement, without rest, using the same equipment - set of repetitions) 1-2 times daily).

13

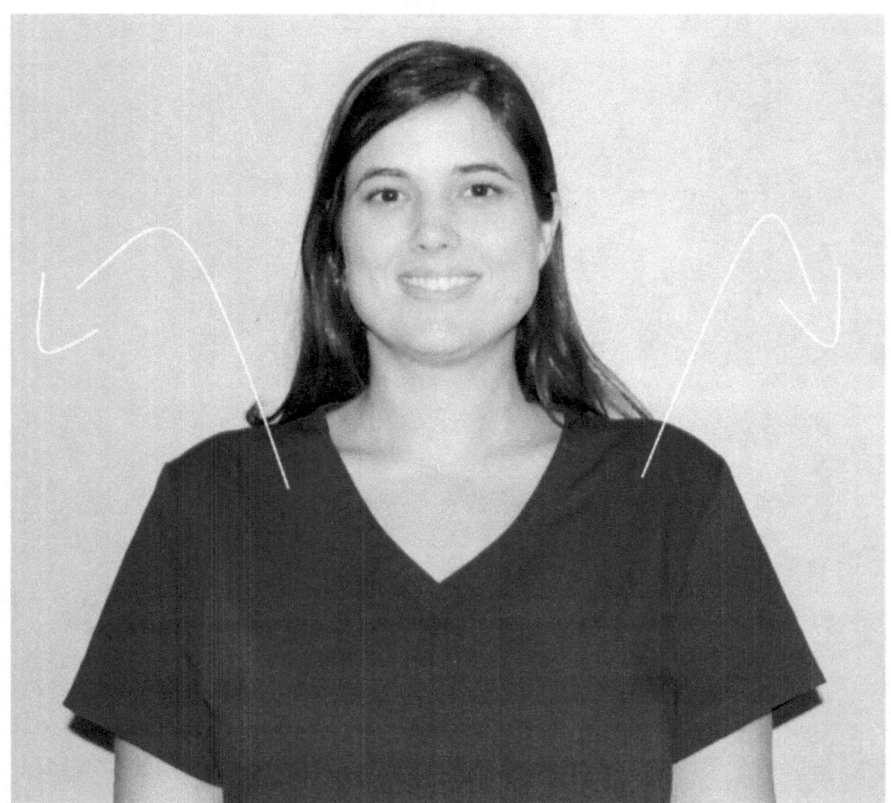

DOORWAY CHEST STRETCH

1. Stand facing a doorway.
2. Keep your elbows bent at 90 degrees with your arms raised to shoulder height.
3. Rest your hands and forearms against the door path.
4. Lean forward slightly causing a stretch of the chest muscles.
5. Hold this position for 5 to 10 seconds to start and gradually work up to 20 to 30 seconds.

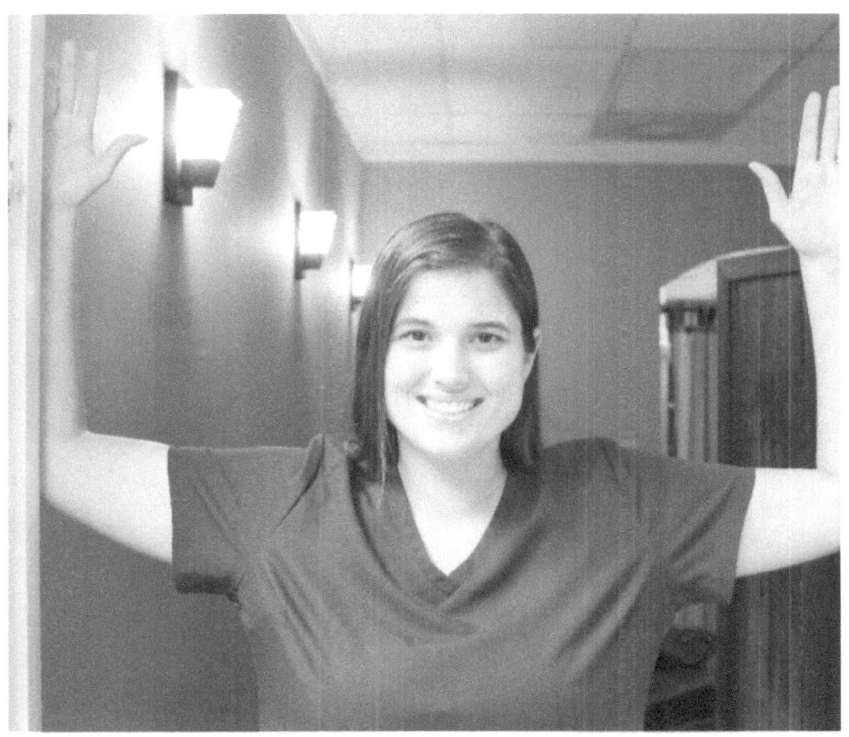

ELBOW ROWS

1. Attach your elastic exercise band or pantyhose to a doorknob or railing.

2. Hold the ends in your hands at waist level.

3. Pull back, bending your elbows and squeezing your shoulder blades together, keeping your elbows close to your side and your forearms parallel to the floor.

4. Hold for 3 to 4 seconds, and then return to your starting position.

5. Complete 1 set of 10 repetitions once or twice per day.

ELBOW ROWS

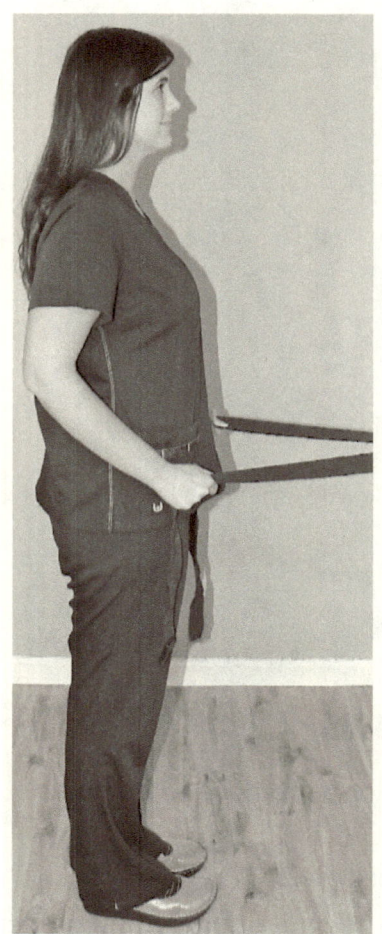 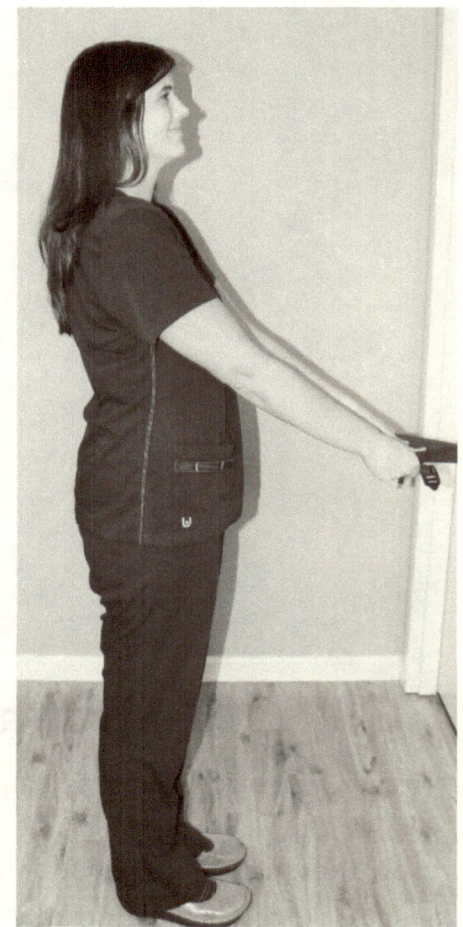

The Physiology of Muscle Development

These exercises may seem too easy to some. To help you avoid the temptation to perform extra sets, I'll explain the physiology of muscle development.

For a muscle to change, it must first be subject to a stimulus, such as weight-resistance exercise. This stress or stimulus results in micro-trauma to the individual fibers (myofibrils) that make up that muscle. When the body repairs these micro-tears, a typical process for muscles, it leads to a stronger and more developed muscle. If the repair process is hindered in any way, the full potential for growth is minimized and the results are disappointing.

When does the repair, process take place? Well, it sure doesn't take place while you are forcing additional sets upon a muscle group that you've already stressed!

Muscle growth and repair occur only when you are resting. No rest equals no growth! This following point is strange, but true. When a muscle has been fully stressed, but not overstressed, rest is the closest thing you can get to using anabolic steroids for muscle growth. The effects are quite similar. So, if you want those muscles to respond to the hard work you put in at the gym or at home, you simply must allow plenty of time for rest, which even includes taking an occasional nap.

Naps are anabolic (tissue building) in nature and work wonders for mental recuperation as well. Rest also means staying away from the gym between workouts. You use these rest days to take care of other life matters or to simply enjoy some leisure time.

Please remember the reason you're doing these stretches and exercises. You're unhappy with past results and are hoping this program will be your answer. It will be your answer if you trust me and allow me to serve as your mentor. Follow the program! Although there are countless things in life that I don't know much about, this topic isn't one of them. This is an area of expertise for me. Please take advantage of that.

Purpose, Plan, and Passion:

You need a compelling purpose to act, one to propel you in the right direction and motivate you to undertake a plan designed to get you what you want.

You need a sound action plan so you have something concrete to work with and strive for, right from day one - a plan that will bring some quick, significant results to show you that you're indeed on the right track.

You need a passion for wellness that will not only fire your imagination so you can see what a future with maximum wellness looks like, but will also inspire you to warmly embrace the continued discipline needed to carry through with your action plan.

Here's the secret:

It is not calendar years, but built-up damage from stress, errant thinking, and lack of crucial movement that are stealing your quality of life!

It starts when you are in your teens and twenties, but you don't notice it. The stress and repercussions keeps building. Then, one day, you "wake up" and begin to see and feel the results. Can grunts, groans, and whimpers be far behind?

No, you can't change your calendar age, but you can resist, or even reverse, years of stress damage if you're not too late. And, the sooner you start, the better the results. It's all about learning science-based secrets for ageless living and shattering the perpetual myths that cloud your vision. But, you do need to recognize the early hints of runaway stress.

Early Hints of Runaway Stress

We get plenty of forewarning about runaway stress - from many directions. Here are some common signs of runaway stress. Even if you haven't experienced some of them yourself, I'm sure they won't surprise you:

☐ You cringe in front of a mirror because of growing bulges, fading muscle tone, or unmistakable signs of "premature aging."

☐ Aches, pains, or a foggy brain have become your closest friends.

☐ You feel tension. You're irritable. You aren't able to concentrate.

☐ You experience dry mouth, teeth grinding, sweaty palms or cold hands, a pounding heart, shallow breathing, chronic headache, low self-esteem, or withdrawal.

☐ Your sleep quality is in the pits and exhaustion rules your day.

☐ You get an upset stomach or urinate frequently.

☐ You have a lowered sexual drive.

☐ Your workouts are, well, not working out!

☐ Tight muscles may cause pain and trembling or you might have nervous twitches.

☐ You know your hormone balances are all out of whack, but you have no idea what to do about it other than suffer.

☐ Your doctor has you worried about the "numbers" from your last physical exam.

☐ Your single greatest weapon for warding off surgery or chronic disease is hope.

☐ You are handling your quality-of-life problems with stimulants, products from a drugstore, and/or the services of "sickness care" professionals.

☐ As a spouse, parent, lover, friend, business owner, employee, student, fitness seeker, or creative worker, your lackluster performance is leaving others out in the cold - and you're not feeling very warm about it either!

It's gut-wrenching for me to see a new patient walk into my wellness clinic who is too far gone for me to help them reverse their pain and ravaged health. Sadly, too much damage has been done for too long. Oh, yes, I can almost always make them more comfortable without pill dispensers drugging them out of their senses, but I just can't get used to serving these troubled ones and their faded hopes. Take Action TODAY!

Train Smarter, Not Harder!

When it comes to resistance training (including weight training), more isn't better. Time and again, I witness individuals spending hours in the gym, five to six days a week, and performing marathon numbers of sets in the futile attempt to gain muscle and body tone. I did that for a full year with NO RESULTS and got very frustrated.

Few people seek competent advice for using resistance training to grow muscle mass or develop better body tone. They do not personally research the methods they use, or even try random changes to see if they can stumble across a better workout.

If you've been seeking advice on exercise routines, I commend you. However, if you're getting your advice from popular muscle magazines - both the male and female versions - you've probably already discovered that most of them follow the - more is better concept? You have read that so-and-so pro bodybuilder or fitness queen performs four different exercises at five sets apiece per body part (for example, the chest). You think, - Well gosh, if it works for him or her, it will surely work for me! Sorry.

With the possible exception of athletes using performance-enhancing drugs, the more-is-better approach leads to overtraining, which is the number one reason body shapers and bodybuilders fail to progress. Performance-enhancing drugs often get results for very heavy trainers because they allow athletes to recuperate more quickly and efficiently following a stressful workout. These athletes, therefore, don't suffer from the tear-down effects of overtraining (but they may suffer from the side effects of performance drugs).

20

Every once in a while, an athlete blessed with superior genes comes along and is able to get spectacular results from heavy workouts year after year without using drugs. But, it hardly ever happens. And, you're not likely to be one with such superior genes or you'd know it. The general rule is that long-term physique builders who follow persistently heavy workout schedules must resort to stress-adapting drugs if they want superior results. Not a pretty picture. But, knowing what research has shown about the deleterious effects of overtraining, I must even question the results achieved by genetically-gifted athletes. I wonder what kind of results they would have gotten if they had allowed for more recuperation and had trained smarter? Would they have been able to achieve even better results if they had spent less time in the gym and more time resting? I think so.

Actually, I'm confident that they would have at least achieved the same physique while cutting the time spent in the gym in half. This extra time could certainly be better spent with your friends and family. What good is a dynamite exterior without an interesting, mature, capable, loving interior to go along with it?

Remember, I am just helping you to have better posture not to look like my favorite childhood character, Incredible Hulk.

Action Item:

Pick one or two simple habits you can adopt in your daily life to improve your posture.

1) _____

_____

_____

2) _____

_____

_____

SIGNATURE: _____

DATE: _____

Chapter 3

R-ELAX

The second letter of my B-R-E-A-T-H system is *R for Relax*. So let's relax and take the time to chill out and just breathe!!

Have you ever just sat and listened to yourself breathe? Did you know that breath channels energy and vitality? Have you ever noticed that when you are stressed or anxious your breathing is shallow? How about when you are relaxed and not worrying? Have you noticed your breathing is deep and full when you are free of stress and anxiety?

Breathing is one of those automatic body functions that is easily taken for granted. Our breathing patterns are actually quite revealing. Often when we need to feel centered, we stop and breathe deeply. Shallow breathing is a way of life for many people. It causes a limited amount of oxygen to reach the bloodstream and can result in fatigue, gas, insomnia, muscle cramps, and feelings of anxiety and panic.

Knowing how to relax and neutralize stress is one of the keys to being happy and living a long, healthy life.

When we breathe deeply, fully, and completely, we counteract the stresses of modern life and calm our mind and spirit. Breathing not only oxygenates the body's 100 trillion cells, it also releases carbon dioxide waste material from each cell.

Smooth, deep diaphragmatic breathing improves blood circulation, gently massages internal organs, promotes elimination of carbon dioxide, strengthens heart and lungs, and promotes deeper sleep patterns.

The next time you find yourself in a stressful situation, sit back and allow yourself time to breathe. Clear your mind, evaluate your body response, and allow yourself time to relax and center yourself.

Half of my office is designed to help you relax. After you receive an upper cervical correction at my office, you go back into my resting suite and lay down to deep breathe. We play soothing music and diffuse essential oils. Our patients love that time, and they use it to relax and allow their bodies to heal.

In fact, I find multiple patients falling asleep and telling me it was their best part of their day. Extra sleep and relaxing is a critical component of healing. Millions of people throughout the world don't get enough rest and sleep. This is a major health problem, and people are tired all the time. I recommend getting 6-8 hours a sleep at night. I also recommended going to bed before 10 pm every night. I heard from multiple doctors that the hours before midnight are most valuable for healing because of the energy of the earth and sun. Have you ever been up late past 1 am and then regained more energy and can't go back to sleep? I have done that multiple times.

The best position to sleep is in on your back with pillows under your knees and a small neck pillow. If possible, sleep with your legs and arms straight and slightly out to the sides. Also, make sure the pillow is not too big to cut off some of your air supply. I have had to correct many spines because of the way people twist and turn in their sleep. Sleep position is crucial to keeping the right posture. Lastly, make sure you clean your pillow case often; as otherwise, you will be breathing lots of dust and bacteria from your head.

According to posture expert Dr. Steven Weiniger, "Diaphragmatic breathing is also called breathing from the belly. A good, deep, cleansing breath should originate from the belly – not the chest."

Place a hand on your belly and the other on your chest. Take a deep breath in. The hand on your belly should rise as your diaphragm fills with air. The hand on your chest should stay still. If you feel the hand on your chest rise with each breath, you have work to do! Chest breathing means shallow breathing and leads to stress, shortness of breath, dizziness, and a higher level of anxiety.

I had to learn how to relax when I started to have an asthma attack, which is the scariest thing on earth. It's like being a fish out of water, or like having thousands of bricks on your chest.

I also learned the Bradley method when I had my kids all natural at home. Yes, that is right. I had all three of my kids at home with no drugs!! I was able to use this technique and have less pain and more bondable memories with my precious babies. The Bradley method of childbirth is natural childbirth, coached by a partner, and my husband Scott was a pro after our first-born Noah's birth. This method helped me to focus on relaxation with my breathing, to reduce my pain, and to have a memorable, unmedicated birth. Another technique I used while being in the most pain of my life was of course, BREATHING. It helped me tremendously. As soon as I focused on breathing and counting, I was able to deal with pain much better. For example, when my contraction would start, I would start counting till it ends (let's say 30 seconds). By next contraction, I knew already that the pain would stop in about 30 seconds, in 15 seconds, 10 seconds, 5,4,3,2,1. And then pain was gone.

While counting, I used some breathing exercises as well: 2 short inhales and one long exhale worked best for me. These two components helped me to survive mentally and physically through my pain.

Keep in mind that what may work for one person may not be helpful for other. It is important to try as many methods as possible to find the best one that fits your personal needs.

Your mental preparation is the key to success if you want a stress free and joyful birth.

Action Item:

Pick one or two simple habits you can adopt in your daily life to improve your relaxed state.

1) _____

_____

_____

2) _____

_____

_____

Chapter 4

E-SSENTIAL OILS, HERBS, AND SUPPLEMENTS

The third letter of my B-R-E-A-T-H system is *E for Essential Oils*. Essential oils are a part of my morning and night routine. Read my routines later in the book for more details.

Most people wake up in the morning and use heavy, artificially-scented shampoos and soaps. They put deodorant with aluminum under their arms, which clogs up our lymphatic system. They use dryer sheets with artificial scents to make clothes smell. All these chemicals are toxic and are closing up our pores and not allowing our body to breathe properly. Long-term exposure to chemicals found in hygiene products, cosmetics, sun-block, fragrances, detergents, and everyday household cleaners causes toxin overload. This stresses the liver and adrenals and causes the body to have dis-ease.

Instead of breathing all of those chemicals and toxins, breathe in essential oils and herbs. Be cautious when supplementing these for the first time. Use one product at a time and see how your body responds. Gradually build up the dosage as you get healthier.

Today, I can say that I've been off my breathing machine and my inhaler (both were steroids) for 15 years and my 3 kids have lived a drug-free life because of what I have learned with natural healing. Yippee!!

In addition to their intrinsic benefits to plants and being beautifully fragrant to people, essential oils have been used throughout history in many cultures for their medicinal and therapeutic benefits. Numerous plants have been identified as having antimicrobial, antiviral, or antifungal properties (3,4,5). Modern scientific study and trends towards more holistic approaches to wellness are driving a revival and new discovery of essential oil health applications.

Essential oils are used for a very wide range of emotional and physical wellness. They can be used a single oil at a time or in complex blends depending on user experience and desired benefit. Essential oils are usually administered by one of these three methods: diffused aromatically, applied topically, or taken internally as dietary supplements. I love putting a drop behind my ears and rubbing it on the back of my skull and then on my lymph nodes in the morning and night (see my routines to find out which ones I use). We are always diffusing my office with therapeutic aromas of a variety of essential oils and everyone enjoys the wonderful smells we create. Using essential oils can be both profoundly simple and life changing at the same time.

Essential oils are plant compounds taken from the root, stems, bark, and leaves.

I have over 50 oils in in my house, but here are the top 3 I started with.

Here are the top 3 essential oils I recommend:

1. *Peppermint* oil was the first essential oil I used over 15 years ago. I commonly use it for running noses, digestion, cramps, and tension headaches. It is very invigorating and antiviral. I use it in my morning routine to wake me up.
2. *Eucalyptus* oil is great for soothing the respiratory system. It opens up your sinuses and aids you in breathing.

3. *Melaleuca* also known as Tea Tree oil is antibacterial and aids in helping your body fight infections. It also has purifying properties for the skin and nails. It is also antifungal, insecticidal, and a strong antiseptic (6).

Using the combination of these three in a diffusor will freshen up the air in your house and help you to breathe better. It's easy to clean with essential oils, and they are super safe and effective. I enjoy making my own cleaners so I can reduce harmful toxins in my home.

For more information on these oils and helpful tips, you can go to: www.mydoterra.com/getwellnc

When my Uncle John would come in town he would use some wonderful herbs and make me a tea. I would put a kitchen towel over my head and breathe in the steam for about 30 minutes and then drink the tea.

There are 1,000s of useful herbs on this planet but I use these daily. It was hard to pick the top 10 because God's plants are so useful in so many ways.

If you have never tried any of the following? What are you waiting for? You will be amazed. If you do purchase any of the below, make sure you are getting these herbs in their purest form.

Top 10 herbs:

1. *Turmeric/Curcumin* is one of the most powerful natural anti-inflammatory herbs in the world (7). I have this in my shake every morning. It is very yellowish orange and stains, so don't get it on your clothes.
2. *Cinnamon* helps stop the growth of bacteria and fungi in the body and may help to increase brain function. It also reduces blood sugar levels in diabetics and helps to lower cholesterol.

As for antioxidants that help fight dis-ease, cinnamon ranks at the top of my list. Every morning I put fresh cinnamon in my morning apple cider vinegar drink. Not only does it taste fantastic, it can relax the tracheal muscles in the lungs. Later in my book, look for my morning and night routines.

3. *Ginger* is in the same family as turmeric. Ginger is the spice of my life. I love it in everything. It makes our smoothies and meals taste so good and it aids in relieving nausea. It was very helpful during pregnancy with the morning sickness days (8). It is also very anti-inflammatory (9). Next time you are making a smoothie, just throw in a little ginger root. I also like making a ginger tea. Peel the root and dice a one-inch slice into 15-20 pieces. Steep in boiling water for about 30 minutes, and enjoy. I like adding some lemon or lime and a dash of honey for a little extra zing.

4. *Plant digestive enzymes*- specifically the pineapple enzyme, Bromelain. It is great in aiding in digestion, supporting immune function, and reducing inflammation. Bromelain is very helpful for people that have chronic sinus issues and has a long history of use as a remedy for sinusitis. Recent clinical trials have found positive benefits in children with sinusitis using bromelain (10,11). These enzymes help break down the food so you can absorb the nutrients from the food you are eating, so taking them before you eat is best. Also, eating raw veggies provides these essential digestive enzymes and you will have less chance of food reactivity. There are also great green (fruit and veggie) drinks that you can consume daily to get all the enzymes you need. It is clear from numerous studies that children and adults who consume a variety of fruits and veggies have a lower risk of allergies and associated asthma.

5. *Garlic* may be stronger than an apple when it comes to keeping the doctor away. It is very healing because it's anti-viral, anti-bacterial, and anti-fungal (12). Also, using garlic oil can be helpful when mixing with essential oils eucalyptus and or melaleuca

for ear infections. You can make your own by warming up some olive oil (about 4 ounces if making a big batch) and adding chopped garlic (about 4-5 cloves). Cook on your lowest heat for 30 minutes. Strain the oil in a cloth and add 20 drops of eucalyptus and 10 drops of melaleuca. Store in an amber bottle and use an eye dropper to suction up the oil from the bottle. Place 2 drops in the ear, and massage behind the infected ear every hour or as needed . A warm sock full of salt is helpful as well to comfort the pain around the ear along with a great upper cervical correction to help the infection from the ear drain.

6. *Cat's claw aka Una de Gato* is what my Uncle John would bring in from a Peruvian tree. It is a bark, and it makes a yummy tea when you add Stevia or honey to it. The bark is known for helping reduce the inflammatory response in the body and it was the first tea I was introduced to help my asthma attacks.

7. *Cayenne Pepper* is also in my morning cinnamon apple cider vinegar drink. This wonderful herb is known for boosting your metabolism, relieving joint pain, and preventing allergies!!

8. *Camu Camu* is one of the highest known sources of vitamin C on the planet and has anti-inflammatory properties (13). Uncle John would also bring this powerful fruit from the Amazon jungle. It has 60 times more vitamin C that an orange. It improves respiratory health, energizes the body, and strengthens the immune system.

9. *Maca* root is another herb my Uncle John would bring in. I am so blessed to have him in my life because I have known about these herbs for 15 years. This one, he put in a formula with cacao and it was delicious. It helps with memory, reduces anxiety, and fuels the hormone system.

10. *Graviola* was one of the herbs we were giving mom daily when she was diagnosed with terminal brain cancer. Again, she lived 3 years instead of 3 months, and I know it was because of God's healing plants we were giving her daily along with all of our

prayers. This herb is known for boosting the immune system by effectively inhibiting the growth of bacteria, virus, parasites, and tumor development (14).

Picking my top supplements is hard, but I want you to get the most from your money when you are buying products. It's clear we can't get all of the nutrients we need for optimal body function and wellness all the time. The only way to know what you need and how much you need is to get tested.

Are you being tested properly? This is why I have success with many health disorders. I test my patients and give them what they need based on the testing that is performed. When it comes to your health, search out a doctor that cares and wants you to succeed in your health journey.

Now to my top 10 supplements.

1. *Psyllium seed/husk* for fiber. Why do I say we need to add more fiber? The number one complaint in my office is gut issues. People today are not getting the right amount of fiber. I strive for at least 30 grams a day. According the Institute of Medicine, women need 25 and men need 38 grams per day. When I am analyzing my patients' diet sheets before they start with me, I calculate that they get about 15 grams or less in their diet. Fiber is a great way to help your body remove toxins. Of course, take plenty of water with psyllium because it expands like gel in the intestines. This gel makes you feel full, so it can also help you with your weight goals. It is very high in fiber and cleans the colon. It reduces bloating and gas and also helps lower cholesterol to a healthier level. Fiber is also considered to be vital in eliminating toxins from the body, limiting the stress these toxins place upon the immune system, and helping us to breathe better.

2. *Vitamin D* is very crucial for immune health (15). Yes, vitamin D comes from the sun, so we need to go outside and open our mouths to take all the sunshine in. Some other ways to get vitamin D are cod liver oil and fish. Vitamin D can reduce your risk of getting autoimmune disease. When I found out I had antibodies on my thyroid and my vitamin D levels were low, I immediately starting taking more vitamin D. That blood test I did 2 years ago was a wakeup call for me. I encourage everyone reading this to get a full check up and let a functional medicine doctor like I analyze it. I no longer have symptoms of Hashimotos (fatigue, overweight, constipated, sensitivity to cold, skin dryness, and puffy eyes,) which is an autoimmune disease of my thyroid and I lost 60 pounds over the course of 2 years. After I got my energy back, the first thing that came to my mind was, "I need to write a book." Go outside now if you can, open your mouth to some warm sunshine, and let that little light of yours SHINE!!

3. *Fish oil* with a high amount of EPA/DHA and GLA. These fatty acids reduce the overall inflammatory burden and improve brain function. A 3-year study concluded if a child was supplemented with fish oil from 6 months to 3 years, they had reduced allergy-related coughs (16). These oils also promote normal growth of blood vessels and help repair nerves. Just like the tin man on the Wizard of Oz...grab the oil can and squirt it (take it internally at night before bed) on your joints to keep them from squeaking. I tell this daily to my patients and they get this oily concept. If you are allergic to fish, avoid this, and use flax seed oil instead.

4. *Probiotics* are the good guys (good bacteria) that help combat the effects of the harmful guys (bad bacteria, yeast, and fungus). From the moment we are born, we breathe in microbes from our mom in the vaginal canal. Babies born by cesarean section don't pass through the birth canal and miss out on the benefits from picking up their mom's microbes. Researchers believe that the epidemic increase in asthma, allergies, type 1

diabetes, celiac disease, and obesity are related to disturbances in the micro biome. Microbes help train the immune system (17). We have overused antibiotics and have messed up our gut. I have heard multiple doctors say we need to be on a probiotic for a year to recover from one dosage of antibiotic. Those singe-cell bacterial organisms are so smart and have become antibiotic resistant, but do not let them outsmart you. Remember, the herbs I mentioned above can help fight off those bad guys. There are multiple strains being discovered every time I turn around. I am constantly changing my probiotics. It is good to start on one and change every time you renew your bottle. Even though my kids have never had an antibiotic and were born vaginally, I still give them probiotics daily because of my overuse of antibiotics as a kid. Several strains of probiotics have been shown to limit some allergy symptoms (18). You can also eat and drink probiotic-rich foods that are fermented, like sauerkraut and kombucha. I love making kombucha. My favorite kombucha is made with green tea, ginger, lemon or lime, and strawberries. Um, Um, good!! There is a video on our Facebook page. Like us to continue to get helpful tips. www.facebook. com/getwellnc

5. *Zinc lozenges* are able to directly inhibit the rhinovirus, which can affect our breathing. Zinc is a vital trace mineral involving in over 300 different enzymatic reactions in the human body. Because zinc enhances our immune system, if we don't have enough in our system, we are more susceptible to infections (19). The body can't store zinc, so we need to get in through our diet or as a supplement. How can you check to see if you are deficient? This is the test we do in our office. Metagenics makes a product called Zinc Tally. It is a simple screening method for evaluating zinc status. By placing two teaspoons of Zinc Tally in your mouth, a lack of taste or a delayed taste perception suggests a possible zinc insufficiency. If they fail, we recommend our patients add zinc to their diet and re-check a month later. More information can be found on cweaver.metagenics.com.

6. *Magnesium* is a wonderful mineral the helps relax the bronchial tubes and smooth muscle of the esophagus. I recommend a product called Calm. It is in powdered form and dissolves very well. This product has worked well for my patients with asthma. It calms the nerves down, and helps you to relax so you can breathe.

7. *Monolaurin* is found in coconut oil and is similar to other mono-glycerides found in human breast milk. As we know, a mother's milk is the best for their baby's health. Monolaurin destroys the protective viral envelope and kills the virus (20,21). It also fights off the bad guys like bad bacteria, yeast, fungi, and protozoa. I have been using a product called Lauricidin for over 12 years, and it is my go-to when my family is feeling a little off.

8. *Vitamin E* has been found to reduce the risk of wheezing and eczema in the children at age two (22). It also helps the free radical damage incurred during the inflammatory response.

9. *Quercetin* is a bioflavonoid that is antihistaminic. It is known to stop certain cells from releasing their inflammatory response, and can be very helpful for people who suffer from allergies (23).

10. *N-acetyl cystenine (NAC)* is an antioxidant that increases gluta-thione levels and thins bronchial mucus. It helps liquefy sinus mucous and removes the bad guys out of the body and helps with pain levels. Yay!! Recent data also suggest NAC inhibits the function of eosinophils, immune cells known to be active in al-lergy-induced asthma, as well as the immune-recruiting chemokines expressed by smooth muscle cells of the human airway (24,25). A product that I love and use daily is called natu-ral D-hist from Orthomolecular. It contains Vitamin C, Quercetin Dihydrate, Stinging Nettles leaf, Bromelain, and NAC. A great combination if you struggle with allergies and want a natural D- histamine to help you get through that season.

Your breathing can improve once again if you maintain a clean environment in your house, reduce your stress levels, eat an unprocessed whole foods diet, and use nutritional supplementation and herbs full of antioxidants.

Action Item:

Which essential oils, herbs, or supplements will you adopt in your daily life to improve your breathing?

1) _____

_____

_____

2) _____

_____

_____

Chapter 5

A-LLERGIES

The fourth letter of my B-R-E-A-T-H system is *A for Allergies.* You have to identify, address, and then eliminate the allergens within your body.

I had my first allergy testing when I was 11 because of all of my asthma attacks. The doctors came to the conclusion that I was allergic to basically everything in the environment because I tested positive on all the skin tests they performed. I also tested positive for some foods, like shellfish. My parents had to get rid of the carpet in my room and put plastic on my bed. My parents were running me back and forth to the hospital with asthma attacks. They almost wanted to put me in a bubble for protection.

The worst asthma attack I can remember was when I was 13 years old, and I had lasagna and a big bowl of ice cream at an Italian restaurant. About 15 minutes after eating, my lungs completely shut down, and again, my parents had to rush me to the ER. Ten years ago, I found out when I eliminated dairy from my diet, my breathing got better because I wasn't so congested. Then two years ago, I eliminated gluten from my diet due to finding out about my thyroid autoimmune disease, and my overall health improved.

There are a variety of allergy tests to determine potential IgE, IgA, and IgG-related immune responses. Positive reactions on skin or blood allergy testing can be a helpful way to discover a particular allergen. In the case of food allergies or sensitivities, the best way to confirm a reaction is to do an elimination and then re-challenge test of the food you suspect to be a problem.

All of our new wellness clients do a specific elimination type diet for 30 days, and everyone notices a huge difference when we eliminate the most common food sensitivities. If the patient is not improving within two weeks I suggest getting a food allergy test done. Food sensitivities may be caused by many factors such as stress, infections, overeating, artificial preservatives, additives, molds, pesticides, antibiotics, and environmental pollutants. Unidentified food sensitivities can then contribute to chronic health conditions like including Irritable Bowel Syndrome, Rheumatoid arthritis, headaches, autism, ADD/ADHD, eczema, chronic ear infections, gut absorption issues, insomnia and many others. When we reintroduce a specific food, we do so one at a time, at least three days apart, to check for any kind of reaction. The reaction can be a skin rash, bloating, joint pain, and just feeling tired again. Listen to your body; it will speak to you.

Common food allergies that we do not want you to consume during the elimination challenge are the following.

Corn

Corn has been heavily subsidized and used in every single possible way you can imagine. The SAD (Standard American Diet) is riddled with corn. 75% of your grocery store is CORN. This is the top food that is genetically modified on a regular basis.

Eggs

Another over-consumed product that is highly processed is eggs. Chickens are fed growth hormones, antibiotics, and are kept in cages with no sunlight or roaming unless specified or organic. Eggs are a common sensitivity that most people are unaware of.

Shellfish

Shrimp, Lobsters, Crabs, and Oysters cause the greatest number of food reactions. This allergy is usually developed later in life. I was highly allergic to shellfish. I still avoid it most times but now that my immune system is stronger I can eat it with no reaction.

Soy

Soy is used in nearly every product. It is difficult to get rid of this substance, but we ask you to reduce consumption as much as you can. Hidden or different names Soy uses: Mono-diglyceride, Soya, Soja, Yuba TSF or TSP (textured soy protein). TVP (textured vegetable protein), Lecithin, or MSG. Soy is also very genetically modified on a regular basis.

Tomato

We consume tomatoes regularly and all throughout the year. A high food sensitivity through years of over using it in our diets. This nightshade vegetable can create a lot of inflammation in our body.

Peanuts

Peanuts are found in a large amount of frequently-used products. Nearly 100 Americans die a year from this allergy. Peanuts are usually infested with pesticides unless purchased organic. (Alternatives – Almond Butter, Sunflower Butter).

Dairy

Processed dairy, which includes milk and cheese, is mucus forming and creates inflammation throughout our body. As many as 50 million Americans are lactose intolerant. Not necessary for human consumption. Traces of DDT and toxic "banned" pesticides are STILL found in conventional milk. Alternatives: Almond Milk, Coconut Milk.

Wheat/Gluten

Common examples of wheat are barley, rye, and oat. Like dairy and soy, gluten is in a myriad of grocery products. So beware of aliases such as "flour, spelt, cake flour, couscous, matzoh, matzah, kamut, and graham."

Here are some guidelines. You will be able to add to them out of your own experience and self-education:

- In order to have health like no one else, you have to live like no one else.
- Consider the "big nutritional picture." Evaluate success over time from many perspectives.
- Always return to your core. If you have a cheat, don't let that become the new norm. Don't allow compromises to add up in your fridge or pantry – ALWAYS return to your core.
- Open your mind to healthy foods, such as fruits, vegetables, lean meats, and healthy fats.
- Set small, achievable goals.
- Implement changes that you can live with for the long run.
- Consider your individual needs.
- When your plan doesn't work, don't give up...make adjustments.

Action Items:

Create a new recipe for yourself. Something that is a little challenging for you and a recipe that you have never made before. It should also be something you desire to eat and is very healthy for you! Go to the grocery store and buy all the freshest ingredients you can find. Then go home and put it all together with the utmost care and attention to detail. Sit down with your friends and family with your best dishes and silverware, and savor the flavors and experience of eating that meal you took total responsibility for.

My favorite food is strawberries, and I love making strawberry shortcake. When I needed to make this new recipe gluten, dairy, and sugar free because of my allergies, I thought it was going to be disgusting. It wasn't, and I have made so many other great recipes that taste better and make me feel great. If you need help with recipes, let me know, and I will share a few.

Write a few sentences about how the food smells and tastes. Write about your reflections on the experience of taking personal responsibility for this healthy meal. How did it feel? How do you feel now about yourself in relation to the food? How do you feel about your ability to get things done and make them happen?

_____

_____

_____

_____

_____

_____

_____

_____

_____

_____

Pick one or two simple habits you can adopt in your daily life to improve your eating habits.

1) _____

_____

_____

2) _____

_____

_____

Chapter 6

T-HERMOGRAPHY

The fifth letter of my B-R-E-A-T-H system is *T for Thermography*. Use thermographic analysis to determine if you have any inflammation in your nerves, lungs, and sinuses.

Being a doctor, I wanted to have a diagnostic tool to assist me in finding inflammation and knowing when and when not to correct the spine. Thermography is the best tool to show the physiology of the body's inflamed areas. Full-body thermographic scans for men and women are a valuable tool for preventative health monitoring to assist with the early detection and analysis of abnormal vascular activity, inflammation, and pain throughout the body.

Thermography is a painless, non-invasive screening test that converts infrared radiation emitted from the skin surface into electrical impulses, which are visualized in color on a computer monitor. This visual image is a graphic map of body temperature, and is referred to as a thermogram.

Thermograms show a spectrum of colors, and can indicate an increase or decrease in the amount of infrared radiation being emitted from the body's surface. Since the normal body has a high degree of thermal symmetry, any subtle abnormal temperature asymmetry (which typically accompanies inflammation, infection, injury, or disease) can easily be identified.

The advantage of using this method of early detection is it establishes a baseline for changes in your health to help prevent future health issues. There is no exposure to radiation and no physical contact with the camera. It is completely non-ionizing, safe, and can be repeated as often as required without exposing the patient to risk.

Here is a face shot of me with thermography. Since the book is in black and white you will have to go to my website to see it in color. Thermography not only shows inflammation in the nerve patterns, lungs, and sinuses. We use it for breast health aware-ness. With every thermography we do in our office, we give away Olivia Newton John's breast self-exam kit called the Liv kit. The Liv kit is a tool you can use over your breast to help you easy de-tect breast lumps. Every woman should be doing breast self-ex- 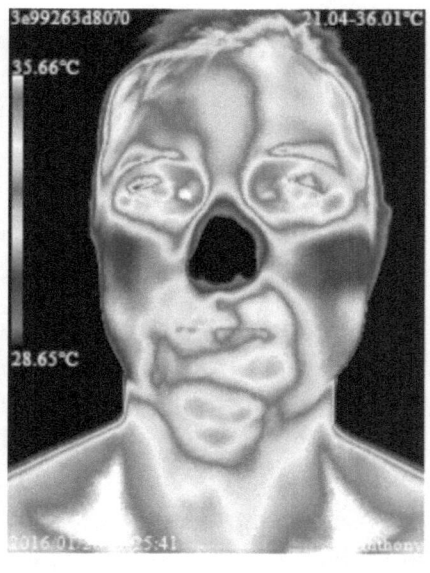 ams. You know your body the best, and the more familiar you get with your body, the more you will know when there's a problem or when something doesn't feel right.

At our office, we give you a plan of action after your thermography results come back in. Here is a sample of some advice we give to our patients.

If your muscles are inflamed in your jaws and neck, we recommend lavender oil on your jaw joint and some neck stretches along with upper cervical care.

If your diaphragm muscle is very tight, we recommend lying with a half foam roll or a towel rolled up under your lower back and deep breathing. We encourage inhaling for a count of 4-8 and then ex-hale for a count of 4-8, and to place one hand on chest and one hand on abdomen to encourage diaphragm breathing. Close your eyes and allow your muscles to relax in the body. The goal would be 6-10 breaths per minute for 10 minutes a day.

Another relaxing technique is soaking in an Epsom salt bath one to two times a week.

If the thyroid is showing cold or very hot patterns, we recommend getting some blood work done for a full thyroid evaluation.

If the thermography shows sinus congestion, we recommend using melaleuca, peppermint, and eucalyptus essential oils behind both ears and doing this massage technique. You can dilute pure essential oils with carrier oil. 1/3 essential oil, 2/3 carrier oil, and put it in a handy roller bottle.

Massaging the sinuses and tissues can help relieve pressure and drain the mucus-filled sinus cavities. Don't get the oils in your eyes when doing this massage. Keep your eyes closed, and use your thumbs to apply the right amount of pressure (pressure that doesn't cause intense pain) starting at your frontal sinuses on your forehead and rub in a circulate motion 10-15 times. Then rub between the eyes and massage in a circular motion around the eyes for 1-2 minutes. Then apply pressure under your cheek bones starting at your nose and going towards your ears. Apply firm and constant pressure for 1-2 minutes. Lastly, steam some peppermint or eucalyptus tea and take a large kitchen towel over your head and breathe in the steam for 5-10 minutes staying about 15 inches away from pot. Do these routines every hour if needed to help relieve the congestion.

Sometimes the patient may need a nasal-specific technique performed. Especially those like me, who had a fall to my face. Accidents and injuries to the face and head can cause the bones of the skull to shift and increase the pressure in our skull, affecting our brain and nervous system. My brother had a broken nose from a baseball bat injury as a kid, and was not breathing at all through his nose. I learned this procedure to help him breathe, and then had it performed on myself. It is a way I can adjust the bones of the skull, specifically the sphenoid bone. The procedure is done with a small balloon, which is inserted into each of your six nasal passages and is gently inflated so the passageway can open. This procedure is not the most pleasant, but can be life changing for patients. My brother and some other patients that struggle to breathe through their noses thank me for learning this technique. Most patients notice immediate improvement in their ability to breathe, and I now can fully breathe through my nose.

If the liver and gut is very inflamed, we recommend starting with Colloidal Bentonite and fiber (psyllium seed/husk). On the first night, take 1/4 cup of the bentonite and swish it in your mouth and then swallow. Then continue with 2 tablespoons each morning and night (leave liquid in mouth for one to three minutes like a mouthwash then swallow). Bentonite clay is a natural detoxifer and helps carries heavy metals out of our body. It also kills bacteria and viruses. The clay itself comes from ash taken from volcanoes. The clay can help draw out toxins, thereby improving immunity and reducing inflammation. It also has beneficial trace minerals we need. We also recommended putting the bentonite clay on a cotton ball on inflamed gum sites for 15 minutes a day.

After you have completed 30 days of using the colloidal bentonite, we recommend coconut oil pulling in the morning (http://coconut-oil-pulling.com/). I recommend using 1-3 tsp. of coconut oil and swish in mouth for 3-5 min. Coconut has antibacterial properties and helps to clean the bad bacteria from the mouth.

Other health benefits of coconut and coconut oil include:

☐ Help you lose weight, or maintain your already good weight
☐ Reduce the risk of heart disease

- ☐ Lower your cholesterol
- ☐ Improve conditions in those with diabetes ard chronic fatigue
- ☐ Improve Crohn's, IBS, and other digestive disorders
- ☐ Prevent other diseases and routine illness with its powerful antibacterial, antifungal, antiviral, and antifungal agents
- ☐ Increase metabolism and promotes healthy thyroid function
- ☐ Boost your daily energy
- ☐ Rejuvenate your skin and prevent wrinkles

I also recommend a liver and gall bladder cleanse. Liver cleanse helps balance hormones and removes toxins from the body, which decreases congestion of lymph in chest/breasts. Performing a quarterly detox is recommended to assist the body in clearing toxins and preventing storage of toxins in the body.

The one I do quarterly is called Clear Change by Metagenics and Core Restore by Orthomolecular. My patients are glad I use these easier ones now, because the one my uncle recommended was a 7-10 day fast with just fiber and herbs. That was my very first detox, and was performed when Noah was one, and it was very hard.

More information can be found on cweaver.metagenics.com or my other websites.

For lymph congestion I recommend dry brushing. Dry brushing helps to stimulate the lymph system and encourages removal of toxins. It is performed with a medium soft skin brush where you start at your feet and brush upward towards your heart. Use firm, but not too hard, small strokes in a circular motion. Brush your whole body and dedicate 3-5 minutes. I do it in the morning before I shower and had noticed increased energy because it also helps stimulate blood flow. A rush of energy is always a good thing in the morning. Do not forget to put on a good natural lotion afterwards. Your skin will thank you!

Rebounding is also fun to do for lymph congestion. It does require a small rebounder trampoline. I have a big trampoline in the backyard, so when I am having fun with the kids I am also helping my lymph system- extra bonus points. I recommend performing 15 minutes a day. A modified version would involve sitting and bouncing on an exercise ball for 15 minutes a day. Both are fun and effective.

Another way to stimulate your lymph system is lightly beating on your chest area like Tarzan. Your thymus gland is in the center of your chest and is part of your immune system. So after you dry brush, beat on your chest like Tarzan in the shower. I know you think I am silly but there is a lot of truth in my words. If you really want to go crazy, add peppermint or eucalyptus to your chest. That will wake you up and get you going for the day!

Another great tool I use to boost the blood flow is the bemer mat, benefiting the body's cardiac system, regenerative abilities, and even mental acuity. It is a mat you lay on and it uses Pulsed Electro Magnetic Field (PEMF) sector. Today, the only similarity between PEMF and bemer devices is the electro-magnetic field. However, the bemer doesn't use PEMF as an active agent, but as a carrier for it's unique physical signal configuration. The bemer owns five global patents and it's research has received numerous scientific awards. It enhances: general blood flow, the body's nutrient and oxygen supply, and waste disposal. It also helps with stress reduction and relaxation.

For more information you can go to
http://drweaver.bemergroup.com/en-US.

For Digestion distress I recommend adding 1-2 tbs of apple cider vinegar before meals. If apple cider vinegar is new to you please start with 1 tsp and mix with small amount of water and honey if desired. I also recommend digestive enzymes, increasing your fiber (1 tsp of psyllium seed/husk per day), and probiotics, as I have mentioned before.

Sometimes on the thermography scan, inflammation shows up where the pyloric valve is. Another technique I have found very helpful to patients is call the pyloric valve exercises. The pyloric valve is between the stomach and the small intestine and is located 2" up from your belly button. It plays an important role in digestion because it controls the flow of food. If the valve is not working properly we have all kinds of digestive symptoms, like acid reflux. Remember when I was talking about the fight and flight mechanism. When we feel threatened, our digestive systems shut down or greatly slow down, slowing this valve. Stress can cause all kinds of problems, including digestive issues. To get this valve working properly again, you can do a release exercise.

When starting this release, start slow, breathe deeply, and do several hours after eating in evening. For more details, see pyloric valve release nstructional video at: totalthermalimaging. com go to: for patients: instructional videos: pyloric valve release.

Some of my goals for patients as they follow the above recommendations are as follows:

1. Decrease muscle tension in neck and face to allow proper nerve function
2. Decrease sinus congestion and improve breathing
3. Cleanse digestive system and liver to eliminate bad bacteria and toxins
4. Improve lymph flow through the body
5. Improve digestion to allow proper elimination of toxins and healthy absorption of nutrients
6. Improve posture to decrease tension on spiral cord

Here are my routines: Sometimes with having small kids, our routines get a little off, but keeping the same routine does help reduce stress and chaos. I find worship music helps us stay relaxed and stay in a praise and gratitude mood.

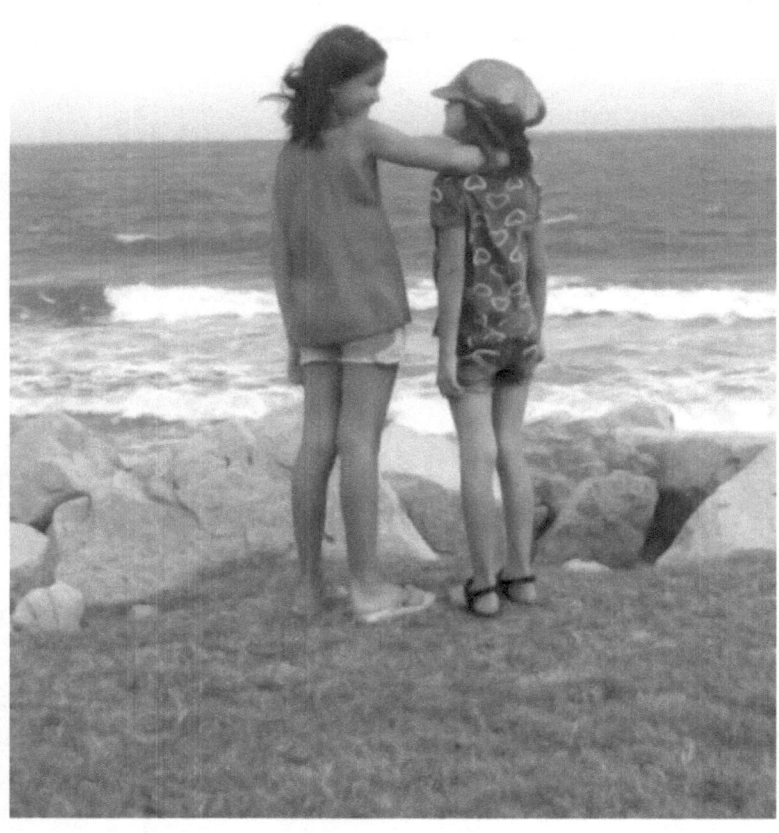

My morning routine	My night routine
1. Have worship music wake me up and do my wall angels.	1. Eat a healthy organic dinner with my family and talk about each other's day.
2. Make my bed because it makes my house feel cleaner.	2. Start a to-do list for the next day.
3. Do my bentonite swish or coconut pulling.	3. Check calendar for tomorrow's appointments.
4. Drink my apple cider vinegar (ACV) *drink.	4. Lay out all of our clothes for tomorrow.
5. Do my turmeric shake with extra fiber and eat an apple a day because it keeps the doctor away.	5. Pack healthy lunches for the kids.
6. Do my dry skin brushing.	6. Take supplements and herbs.
7. Take a shower with my peppermint and eucalyptus oils and do my Tarzan moves.	7. Clean face with organic cleanser.
8. Put natural lotion on.	8. Brush teeth.
9. Get dressed and brush teeth with Doterra's On Guard toothpaste or my homemade one.	9. Put lavender and melaleuca essential oils in my diffuser in my bedroom and on my jaw and neck/lymph nodes.
10. Put my all natural makeup on and SMILE because it is going to be a great day in the neighborhood.	10. Read my Bible.
	11. Do my deep breathing exercises and some yoga stretches.
	12. Snuggle with my husband, Scott, with a big SMILE on my face.
	*ACV Recipe (1 cup of water with 2 tbsp of ACV, a shake of cayenne pepper, 1 shake of cinnamon, and 1-4 grams of powdered vitamin C).

Action Item:

Pick one or two simple habits you can adopt in your daily life to improve your inflammation in your body.

1) _____

_____

_____

2) _____

_____

_____

Chapter 7

H-EAL FROM INSIDE

The final letter of my B-R-E-A-T-H system is *H for Heal from inside*. We must Heal.

We have to forgive ourselves and other people in order to be healthy. I have a good friend who is an oncologist, and he once told me, "Corinne, the cause of cancer is un-forgiveness." We have to forgive ourselves and other people in order to be healthy. The first step in this is confession and receiving the forgiveness and restored fellowship that are the result of that confession (1 John 1:9). There is no doubt that God will bless the pursuit of a passion for Him and will glorify His name through it.

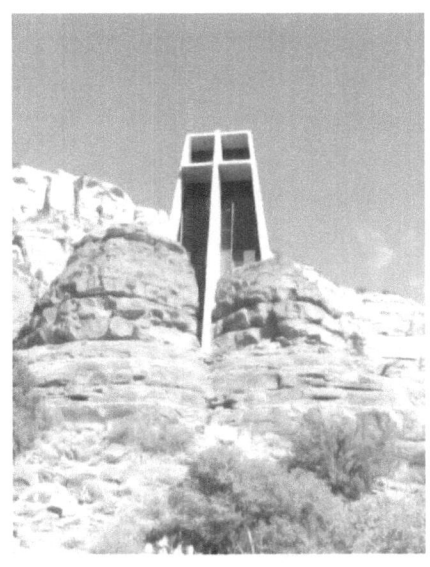

The word forgive comes from a Greek root word meaning "to set free or to let go." I promise I won't start singing from Disney's *Frozen*, "Let it Go, Let it Go!" To forgive you have to decide to give up any urges you have to be angry or resentful. Disown those feelings and walk away from them. Set yourself free and let go and let GOD!

I know it's not easy, but that un-forgiveness is poison filling your body with sickness. So just love instead. Remember, forgiveness is not something we do for other people. We do it for ourselves so we can get well and stay well.

One of my favorite songs from my aunt, Olivia Newton John is Grace and Gratitude. My mom was diagnosed with terminal brain cancer and only given 3 months to live. Even though she still passed away, she didn't live 3 months- she lived 3 years. We shared a gratitude diary, and mom and I would reflect on things for which we were grateful.

Here is a picture of my mom's mom, my sister, and me.

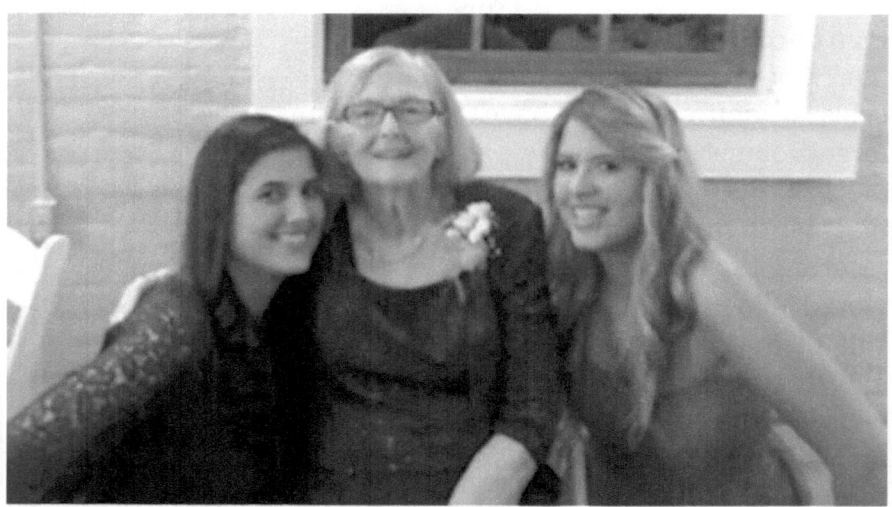

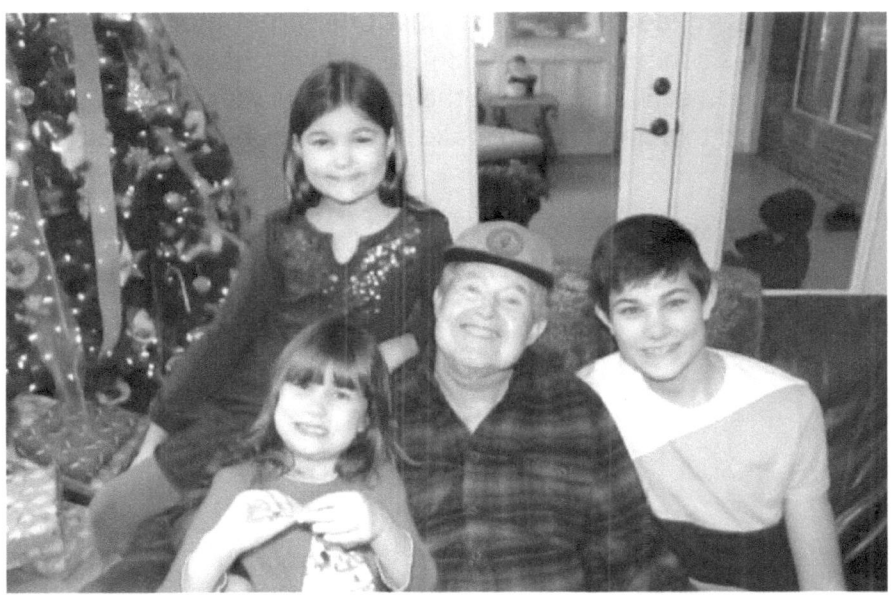

Here is a picture my wonderful grandfather and my kids. His book is very inspiring. It's because of him that I have overcome my fears and become courageous to keep pushing for my dreams and doing whatever it takes for me to make them happen.

Celebrating my dad's birthday is just one of the many things we love to do as a family. I love making birthdays feel special because it is a way you can look back at the marvelous year memories and look forward to a new year to make new wishes become reality.

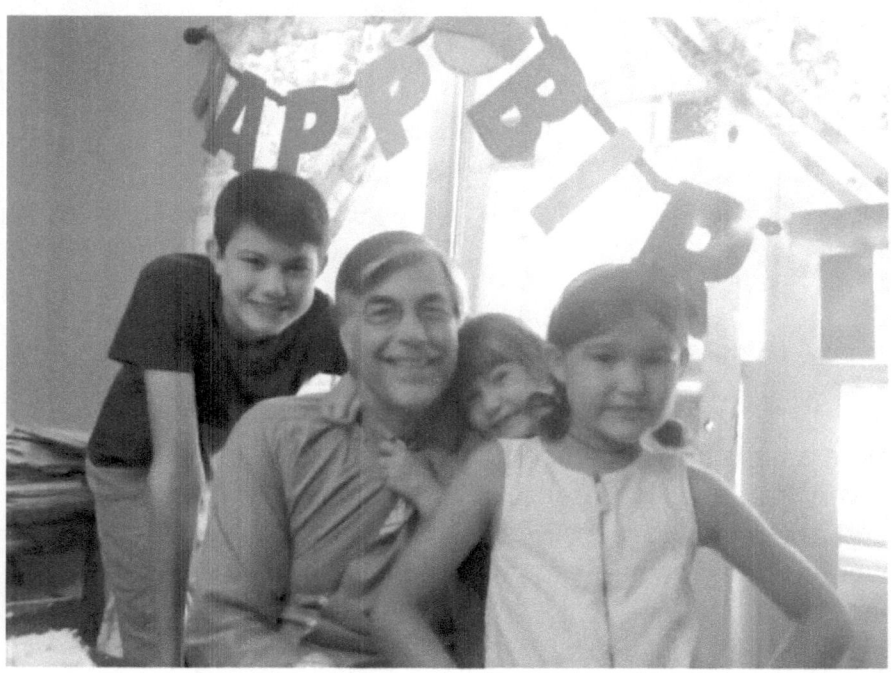

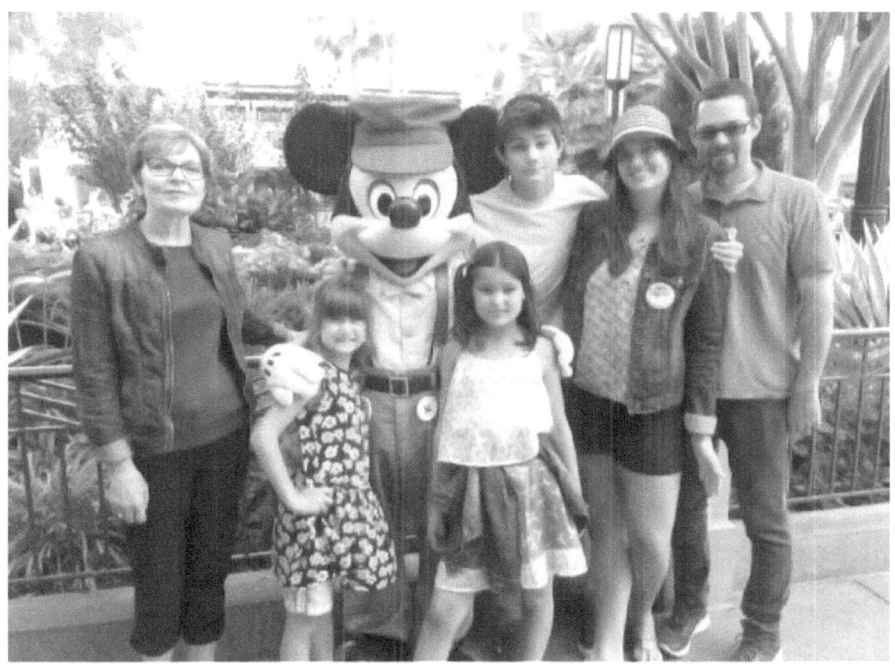

Here is a wonderful example of us being with Scott's mom making dreams come true. As Walt Disney would say it, "If you can dream it, you can do it."

Here is my wonderful wellness team. My list is very long of all the people I am thankful for. Without relationships with family and friends, I would not enjoy the richness of my life.

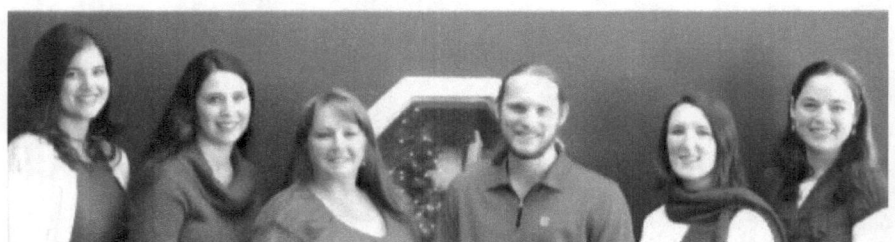

Every day this week, I want to encourage you to write down at least seven things for which you are grateful. Of course, you can write more if you want. This diary mom and I shared is so precious to me. She was thankful for her cancer because it brought us close together, and those memories are truly the best. Take this time to pray, be alone with your thoughts, listening, letting everything external in the world go, and being in peace. "Be still, know that I am God." Psalm 46:10

1. _____

2. _____

3. _____

4. _____

5. _____

6. _____

7. _____

I also want you to take this time to call your mom and /or dad (if you are lucky enough to have them still living on this Earth) and tell them you love them. Tell them how much you appreciate them and how great is to be alive today. Also call your brother(s) and / or sister(s) and tell them how much you appreciate having them in your life. Lastly, call your oldest best friends and tell them how much their friendship has meant to you over the years. This might be the last year of your life or theirs.

My bro and sis at his California wedding.

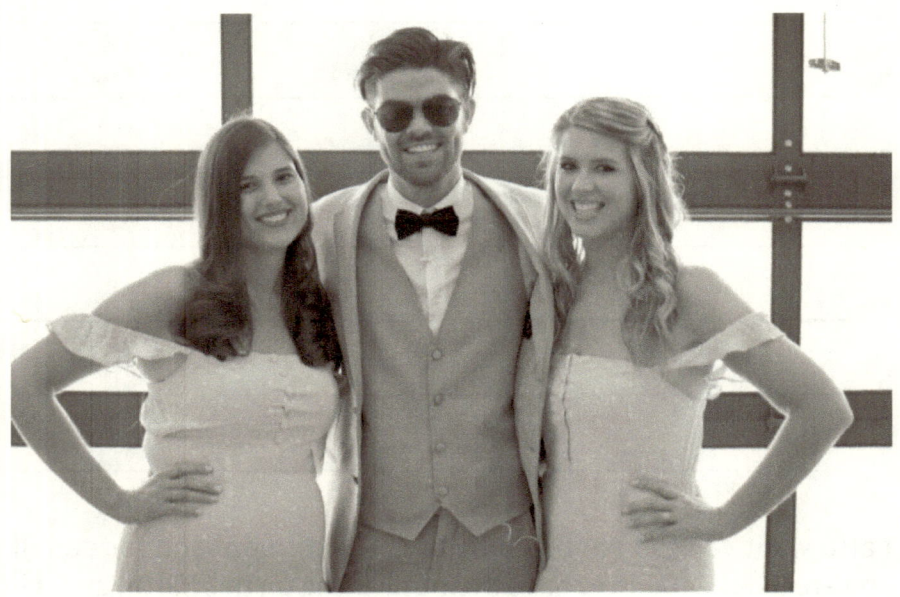

Stephanie, one of my best friends, and I at the Grand Canyon! These moments would have not happened if not planred out. Do a huge favor for yourself and go after your dreams.

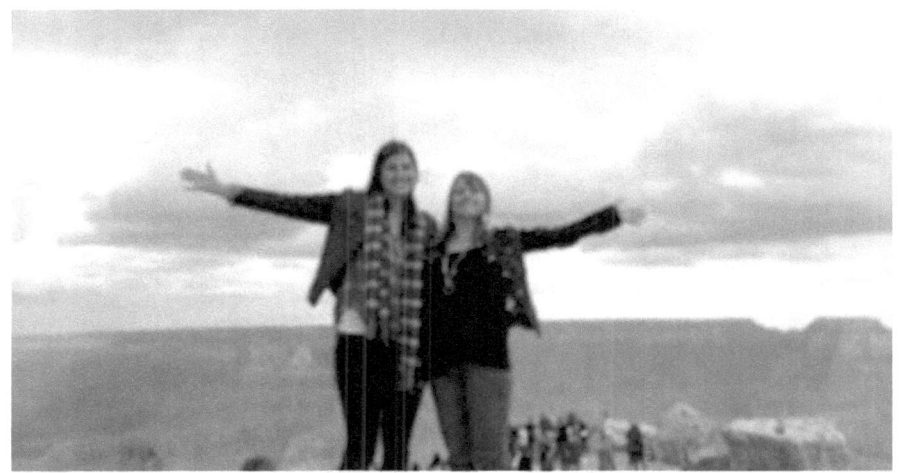

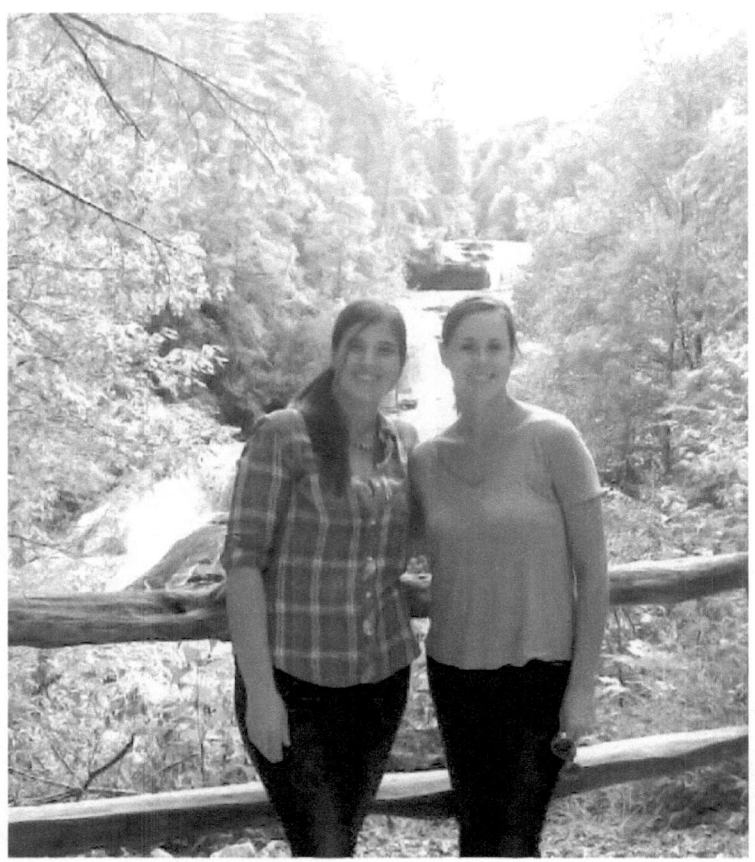

Tiffany, one of my best friends, and I in the mountains by a peaceful waterfall.

Taking a walk with your best friend on the beach or in the woods, or in the mountains by a waterfall is one of the most joyful times you can give yourself.

One of the beautiful memories I have with my mom is when John and Olivia came to visit. John was giving mom amazing herbs in her mouth from the Amazon jungle, and Olivia was singing to her the Grace and Gratitude song and massaging her feet. I can remember that moment being so precious. We have to be grateful for everything we have. Life is too short not to just breathe in the positive light within us.

My mom's favorite movie was the Wizard of Oz. I must have watched it over 100 times. Looking back at that movie, there were some lifelong principles that I use today.

Just like Dorothy in the *Wizard of Oz* had all the power inside her to get home, each of us have that same super-power within us to heal any ailment with our BREATH!!

I was with mom during her last Breath and that moment was the most peaceful experience I have ever encountered because I knew where she was going. I know she is somewhere over the rainbow of heaven looking down and smiling at me with her most beautiful smile.

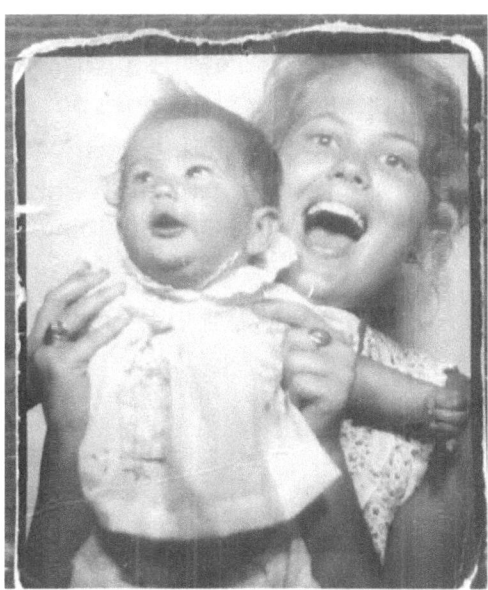

My mom and me.

Here are some wonderful breathing techniques that mom and I would do together when she was fighting to live with cancer and I now do every day.

Enjoy!!

Belly Breathing

The first thing you need to learn to do is what's called Belly Breathing. This is the most basic of the breathing methods we can do anytime, and therefore, is the one you should master before trying out the others. It's very simple, and requires just a few steps:

1. Sit down comfortably, or lay down on a yoga mat, depending on your personal preference.
2. Place one of your hands on your stomach, just below your ribcage. Place the second hand over your chest.
3. Breathe in deeply through your nostrils thinking positive healing thoughts letting your first hand be pushed out by your stomach. You should find that your chest does not move.
4. Breathe out through your lips all the negative thoughts in your live, pursing them as if you were about to whistle. Gently guide the hand on your stomach inwards, helping to press out the breath.
5. Slowly repeat between 3 and 10 times.

You should begin to feel relaxed as soon as you have repeated the Belly Breathing exercise two or three times, but keep going for as long as you feel you need to. After you have mastered this breathing exercise, there are four additional methods for you to try, ranging in difficulty.

4-7-8 Breathing

The method which we call 4-7-8 Breathing also requires you to be sitting down or lying comfortably. Here are the steps you need to follow:

1. Get into the same position as you did for the Belly Breathing exercise, with one hand on your stomach and one on your chest.
2. Breathe in slowly but deeply. Take 4 seconds to breathe in, feeling you stomach move in the process.
3. Hold your breath for 7 seconds.
4. Breathe out as silently as you can manage, taking 8 seconds. Once you reach 8, you should have emptied your lungs of air.
5. Repeat as many times as you need, making sure to stick to the 4-7-8 pattern.

Roll Breathing

If you are looking for a breathing exercise that you can do comfortably sitting down, try the Roll Breathing method. Its aim is not just to relax, but also to encourage the full use of your lung capacity. Beginners are advised to lie down, but after your first time you should find it just as easy to sit and complete this exercise. Follow these steps:

1.Position yourself with your left hand on your stomach, and place your right hand over your chest. Your hands should move as you inhale and exhale.

2.Take a deep breath from your lower lungs; breathe slowly, ensuring that the hand over your chest doesn't move as you take the breath. Make sure you are using your nose to breathe in, and then exhale using your mouth.

3. Repeat the deep breath up to 8 times. On the ninth repetition, once you have filled your lower lungs, take a breath which will move your chest up, as you would normally breathe. This will fill your entire lung capacity.

4. Gently exhale through your mouth, being sure to empty your lungs as you do so. While you exhale, make a small whooshing noise. You should notice that both of your hands are moving back towards your body, as your stomach and chest fall.

5. You should practice this method for between 4 and 5 minutes. When you exhale, you should be able to feel a tangible difference in your stress levels.

Morning Breathing routine

While the above three exercises can be completed whenever necessary, the next method is called Morning Breathing and, as the name suggests, should be practiced once you have woken up. It aims to relax your muscles after a good night's sleep, and will help you to minimize tension for the remainder of the day. Here are the steps to follow:

1. Stand up straight and, slightly bending your knees, bend your torso forward from the waist. Your arms should be hanging close to the floor, limply.

2. Take a breath in slowly, returning to your original standing position. You should look like an inflatable Gumby balloon. Your head should be the last thing to straighten up.

3. Exhale, returning to the position of being bent forward by the end of your exhale. Stand up straight once you have finished, stretching your muscles as required.

Night Breathing Routine

Finally, the Deep Muscle Relaxation technique s the most time-consuming, but can also be the most rewarding for your body. This works best when combined with the Belly Breathing that I mentioned earlier, and is a great way to attain full relaxation. You will exercise each major muscle in turn, but pay most attention to any muscles that are causing discomfort or ache. To start, lie down in a comfortable position and focus on your Belly Breathing, closing your eyes if need be. Then do the following

- To relax your face, knit your eyebrows together and release.
- To relax your neck, tilt your head down towards your neck, and push your chin to your chest, then release.
- To relax your shoulders, make a shrugging motion, then release and roll.
- To relax your arms, push both arms away from your torso, stretch them out, and then relax them by your side.
- To relax your legs, point your toes as far away as they will stretch, and then relax.

All of these stretches should be conducted at the same time as the Belly Breathing we covered earlier. Breathe long and deep, and take your time with each stretch. I enjoy doing this with soothing ocean sounds.

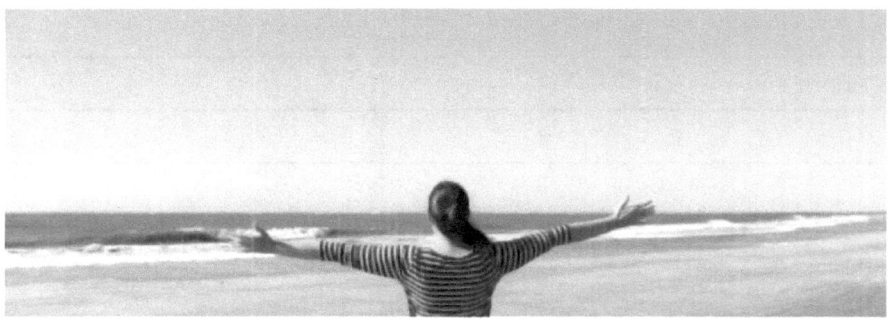

Imagine yourself walking on the beach and you come across a unique bottle. You pick it up and rub on it. Suddenly a genie appears and grants you three wishes.

What would your three wishes be?

1) _____

2) _____

3) _____

Ideally all of us want and desire to be happy.

So I ask you, what makes you happy?

_____

_____

_____

_____

_____

_____

_____

_____

_____

_____

_____

_____

_____

Not that I have already obtained all this, or have already arrived at my goal, but I press on to take hold of that for which Christ Jesus took hold of me. Phil. 3:12

Action Items:

Sometimes, I have found some of my patients can't forgive themselves. This week, I want you to actively make the choice to be kind to yourself. Show compassion for yourself at least one time each day, and make notes about each time and how you felt. Once you get comfortable with loving yourself, it will be easier to show love to others.

DAY 1

_____

_____

_____

DAY 2

_____

_____

_____

DAY 3

_____

_____

_____

DAY 4

_____

_____

_____

DAY 5

_____

_____

_____

DAY 6

_____

_____

_____

DAY 7

_____

_____

_____

Now make a conscious effort to be kind to one person each day this week and let me know how it turns out. Have fun, and get comfortable with getting out of your comfort zone.

Chapter 8

MIGRAINES DISAPPEAR

Jamie fell in her house when she was taking off her shoes on March 14, 2008. She was 8.5 years old and in the 2nd grade. She had a 14-month-long migraine due to the concussion she had with the fall.

Before meeting Dr. Weaver, she tried adult migraine meds, in-hospital IV treatment, physical therapy, massages, swimming/running. None of these treatments worked.

Jamie had a daily headache and her eyes were always dilated since her fall. Dr. Weaver took spinal x-rays, and they reminded her mom of a question mark.

After her first upper cervical correction, the headache went away and the eyes were no longer dilated.

After a few months of care, a recheck of x-rays was performed. Her entire spine was back into alignment without an adjustment to the rest of her back.

Braces went on in January 2010 and the headaches and dilated eyes came back. With a quick appointment with Dr. Weaver and an orthodontia adjustment to take the pressure off her teeth, her headaches were gone and her eyes went back to normal. Then, Jamie sustained another concussion. Dr. Weaver's office was the first place her mom brought her because she learned from the last experience and didn't want Jaime to suffer like she did before.

Earlier, I mentioned how your eyes can be dilated from activating your sympathetic nervous system. In this case, her concussion caused inflammation in her brain and vagus nerve, which lead to Jamie's headaches and her pupils being dilated.

Jamie got under upper cervical care at my office and saw improvements with her first correction. She was glad someone told her to come to my office and her mom listened.

Upper cervical care is a form of chiropractic and is defined as the discovery and removal of the vertebral subluxation, which is interference that is taking place in your central nervous system (CNS). It is important to recognize that our CNS is the master controller of our entire body and it directly correlates to our ability to function and exist. If our body is not getting the information it needs from our brain, our body will be at dis-ease. I like to refer it to dis-ease rather than disease. The idea is to choose not to empower health issues by focusing on a particular ailment. The term dis-ease simply means lack of ease or harmony within the body.

People, who are suffering from dis-eases like allergies, asthma, headaches, etc., are often living subluxated, but when we provide these individuals with an upper cervical correction, we are able to remove the interference, and often, the symptoms associated with these conditions may dissipate. In addition, patients who are under regular upper cervical chiropractic care actually prevent these situations from impeding upon their lives.

What is Subluxation?

Maybe you are wondering where a "subluxation" comes from. It is the direct result of everything that we do. Lifestyle stresses, perceived as either positive or negative, result in nerve interference, which needs to be addressed. For example, during the holiday season, many people tend to consume a substantial amount of food and alcohol and also spend more time with family (which some would consider stressful). What I have seen is that after the holiday season, people typically get sick, which happens to be caused by a subluxation. The food, alcohol, and family represent lifestyle stresses, even if they are labeled as positive, because our body is extremely sensitive to external factors. This is why upper cervical chiropractic care needs to be an essential component of your life, and something that we encourage your entire family to consider.

Upper cervical doctors are different than other chiropractors. We use specific laser-aligned x-rays to help us determine how to correct your spine. In order to perform the right correction to the upper spine and head, x-rays need to be performed to measure and examine your unique anatomy.

Another tool I use is thermography, which I explained earlier. I use paraspinal thermography (heat reading) to establish a pattern the nervous system is making and monitor the readings each visit. I believe you should hold your spinal correction as long as possible so I only correct your spine when your body shows objective findings from the thermography that a correction is needed. If I find I am correcting your spine every visit I see you, it is a sign that your lifestyle is creating an imbalance, and I will need to review some lifestyle changes with you so you can heal. Healing starts when you are holding your correction and your brain-to-body communication is 100% flowing.

As an upper cervical doctor, I don't snap, twist, or pop the upper spine. I use a gentle realignment procedure to bring the head and neck into better balance.

At my office, we take the upper cervical chiropractic lifestyle to a level where it becomes REAL for you. Not only do we offer the upper cervical correction, we take into account your entire body and the lifestyle choices that you make when developing customized protocols for you to follow. These combine individualized programs with tips on fitness, nutrition, and stress relief.

Chapter 9

LIVING WITH LESS ANXIETY

isa had an overactive thyroid that could not get stabilized. She had nervousness, anxiety, lack of concentration, fatigue, weakness, reflux, high cholesterol, leg pain, and low back pain.

She was constantly sick with flus and viruses. She missed a lot of work.

She tried general chiropractic, physical therapy (with orthopedic specialist,) and muscle/pain relaxing medications.

Upper cervical care and seeing Dr. Weaver allowed her to improve her health. Her thyroid and cholesterol numbers stabilized and improved. She now has more energy, better concentration, better attitude, less anxiety, less pain in legs, less pain in low back, and more mobility in her neck. Her x-rays showed an improved cervical curve and a straighter spine.

So many people deal with anxiety on a daily basis. I did too. I had anxiety not knowing when I was going to be in a situation where I couldn't breathe. Having asthma caused me to have anxiety attacks. Now, knowing how to breathe with ease is a huge blessing I don't take for granted. I am so thankful to know how to breathe during stressful times, and my purpose with this book is to educate and motivate you to do the same.

One way to monitor your stress is to check your adrenal function. Adrenal salvia testing, the iris contraction test, and postural low blood pressure are ways to monitor your adrenal function.

Adrenal salvia testing

These days, it is generally accepted that saliva cortisol testing is the most accurate test, as it gives a better estimate of the cortisol levels within your cells, where the hormone reactions are actually taking place.

Here's another important thing to know about cortisol testing. Taking a single measurement, or even a 24-hour average, is not enough. The best cortisol tests take 4 individual samples at various points of the day and then map your cortisol levels over the course of a 24-hour cycle. Our cortisol levels vary dramatically, starting high when we wake up, and then tapering off until they reach their lowest point late at night. This usually represents something like an 80% drop, which is perfectly normal.

The Iris Contraction Test

First described by Dr. Arroyo in 1924, this test measures the contraction of the iris in response to repeated exposure to light in a dark space. In those with weakened adrenal function, the theory goes that the iris will be unable to maintain its contraction for long.

To conduct the test, sit in a darkened room in front of a mirror. Take a flashlight and shine it across your eye, from the side of your face. In a hypo-adrenal state, your pupil will not be able to hold onto its contraction for more than 2 minutes and thus will begin to dilate despite light repeatedly shining on it. In those with healthy adrenals, the contraction should last much longer.

Postural Low Blood Pressure

When we stand up, those of us who are in good health experience an almost immediate rise in blood pressure. In contrast, adrenal fatigue sufferers will see no change in their blood pressure, or even a slight fall. In very general terms, a larger drop in blood pressure signifies a more severe case of adrenal fatigue and your body is crashed out.

This is a very simple test to do at home. Use your regular blood pressure monitor and check your blood pressure while lying down. Then stand up and conduct the test again.

To help you be less stressed at my office, you go to our nice resting suite to relax after you receive an upper cervical correction. This suite is cell phone free, and I play relaxing music to help your body to relax. I have encouraging words on the walls to help my patients think positive thoughts as they BREATHE!!

Chapter 10

NO MORE BLOOD PRESSURE MEDICATION

Lori was sick for 14 months and only 38 years old. She suffered from high blood pressure, fatigue, and many other symptoms.

After Dr. Weaver did the tests that were necessary, she found what was causing Lori's blood pressure to be high. After starting her wellness program, her blood pressure dropped. She got off all her medicines because she was now healthy. She now knows how to eat better with the Wellness U classes (Dr. Weaver's Wellness University) and the information given to her. This curriculum includes nutrition, simple cooking techniques, detoxification, organic shopping on a budget, fitness, exercise, stress management, and herbal-o-logy (natural herbs and home remedy solutions). The supplements were a huge help to her recovery. Her energy is now back, and now she can enjoy her life with her kids.

Lori was surprised how quickly her energy came back and how quickly her blood pressure went down to normal. She now thinks differently when she is planning her meals for her family.

Many moms just like Lori come to my office. As moms, we take care of everyone else besides ourselves. I have been there too. I realized if I don't take care of myself, I am no good for anyone else. You can't force someone to take care of themselves. They have to choose to quit smoking, exercise, and eat healthy.

If we are not constantly working to improve ourselves, we do not remain the same. Rather, we deteriorate in response to the laws of time. If we're not going forward; we're going backward. Staying the same isn't an option for us, though many live as though they have such an option and fight hard for it. (Hint: It doesn't work.)

So, how do we begin to make these changes? How can we guarantee that next year brings more pleasant circumstances and rewards than the last few? The answer is really basic and uncomplicated. Though there are uncommon exceptions, the choices we make in life determine the outcome. We reap what we sow. Start making better choices and forming better habits...one day at a time. Remember to always consider the long-term implications, not just the immediate gratification. Keep in mind, every day we are forming habits.

Periodically, all of us have had to deal with bad habits. It seems that once we acquire them, they take up shop and move into our subconscious mind on a permanent basis. We know that bad habits lead to no good, yet we continue to allow them to rule over our God-given decision-making abilities. Why is this so?

Habits are formed within the neurological framework of the mind. Just as a stream of running water cuts pathways into the earth, habits shape neuronal paths within the nervous system. Once these paths have formed, it's easier to follow the learned behavior than to change it. The good news is that all habits can be changed the same way they were created ... one day at a time. It takes 4 to 6 weeks for these neuronal paths to form, and the same amount of time to revise or interrupt them.

Can you take 6 weeks out of your approximately 4,160 weeks of life to break bad habits? You can, if you know how to replace them with habits that bring results. Remember, you're more likely to continue something if the outcome brings pleasure. Doubly so if you're simultaneously removing pain.

You must adopt one important behavior if you're to achieve continued success in letting go of nasty habits: DON'T FOCUS ON GETTING RID OF THEM! Don't make the mistake of thinking bad habits such as smoking, excessive coffee drinking, or frequent sugar infusions are friends or comforting partners in life. Think on POSITIVE BEHAVIORS and make the transformation slowly.

Pause for a moment and breathe in deeply 7 times. Yes, take this time right now and breathe. First, take a deep breath and feel your chest inflate with positive energy full of refreshing oxygen. Hold this breath for a couple of moments and reflect on the things you are grateful for. Then exhale and expel all that is negative from your body, visualize negativity, dis-ease, and addictions leaving your body with your out breath. Now repeat 6 more times and enjoy this moment in time.

If a goal is important to you, only share it with one or two close, trusted friends. Ee sure they have given support to your past dreams and goals. Such encouragement can help.

The Breath of Freedom!

As you start to let go of old, worn-out habits that have kept you stagnant for years, you begin to feel a sense of freedom. It's really quite beautiful to feel that you're actually in control of your future. It's like waking up on a bright, fresh spring morning after a good night's rest with no commitments for the day! When you finally replace those negative habits with positive ones, nothing will keep you from seizing and taking advantage of your wonderful life.

Aside from the obvious health benefits, what else have you been missing by remaining the same? In your mind's eye, take a good look at what you've been missing - since it's going to be one of the goals you're going to move toward. Might it be a positive self-image? With an improved self-image comes self-respect and discipline. With self-respect and discipline comes the desire to take on new challenges in life. As you take on new challenges, you gain confidence. Then, along with confidence, arises the new habit of projecting your positive best for the benefit of others. Positive thoughts and behavior toward family, friends, and co-workers lead to others step out of their comfort zones and take control of their lives as well as supporting your efforts. It's amazing how all these benefits accrue and follow on the heels of each other just by starting along a pathway that embraces a positive self-image!

If you're like most other people, you consider it a major problem to find the time in your hectic schedule to change your behaviors. Here's a little secret. Time is always a problem (real or imagined) no matter who you are or what you do for a living!

Lack of time is the flimsiest of all excuses, but it's the easiest, most convenient one to use. Many people find time to take care of themselves and exercise while working 40 hours per week. Others who work two jobs and 70 hours per week also find the time. In truth, there is no time to find. There is only time to allocate. And, we allocate based on our chosen priorities. This all boils down to choice. Don't fool yourself with the time excuse. You're the one who loses.

You may have heard me say that health is our most valuable asset. My family is most important to me, and is the reason I must make my health my number one asset. Deny yourself proper care today, and both you and your family pay the price of neglect tomorrow.

Over the past 12 years, I've had the opportunity to work with thousands of patients and have seen countless families devastated by serious illnesses and debilitating diseases affecting their spouses, parents, or grandparents. Most of these conditions have been brought on by inactivity and obesity and, therefore, can usually be avoided. If you consider yourself a supportive human being and you want to place your loved ones above everything, then you absolutely need to rethink your attitude toward reordering your time priorities and caring for yourself. Remember, your time with the Wellness U program will be well spent because it induces changes that bring greater joy of life not only to you, but to your family as well. It's the joy of being able to be there, with full personal resources, for those who you love and who depend on you!

What's another reason to take care of you? Renewed health brings renewed energy. This means you soon find that you're accomplishing more work, completing more activities, and catching up on past projects in less time and with less stress. You'll be amazed to find how much you can do in a day when you have enhanced energy and enthusiasm to work with.

If you still question your ability to move into action and make something happen with the time you have, here's something to consider. Celebrate the gift of your body. And care for that gift wisely! Start by developing good habits and crowding out the bad ones.

Wellness is 95% Self Care: Don't Forget to Take Care of You!

There you go again, always taking care of someone else- your children, your aging parents, a sick relative or friend, an out-of-work sibling. But, what have you done for you lately?

While it's commendable to want to help others, charity begins at home, they say. "At home" here means taking care of you because, if you don't do that, you certainly can't help anyone else.

A holistic approach to taking care of you incorporates caring for your physical body, emotions, intellect, and spiritual self from a wellness outlook.

Chapter 11

BREAKING OLD HABITS

Sammee being 68 years old was overweight, tired, and not that knowledgeable about sugars and additional chemicals in food. She learned to eat whole foods and read food labels.

When she joined Dr. Weaver's team, she learned to be accountable to someone, lose weight, and be as healthy as she can be. During this time, she was able to get off her prescription drugs.

She learned to be more aware of her body and the way it functioned. She also learned how proper nutrition can help keep her healthy. Learning this good information has helped her to listen to her symptoms and understand how her body is all connected and affects itself. She now has more energy and endurance throughout the day. She is amazed by how much she can eat and still maintain good weight, just by eating healthy foods. Even though it's hard work to stay healthy, it is worth it. She was intrigued by the before and after positive results seen on Dr. Weaver's extensive blood work panel.

Anyone can learn how to eat healthy. Sammee is just one of the many I have helped get off her medications. She was able to get off her meds because she was dedicated to learn and take action for her own health. Going over her comprehensive blood report helped her to stay on track because she wanted to see positive results when doing the second blood analysis. Accountability was also a key to her success. Here are some helpful food tips that we share in our office that you can start doing too.

Buying Organic is one way to help you stay away from more chemicals. The third most common mistake we make when we breathe.

Here are more reasons to buy Organic.

Produce:

- ☐ Grown without synthetic fertilizers or irradiation
- ☐ Is not genetically engineered or modified
- ☐ Grown without chemical pesticides
- ☐ Grown in high quality soil
- ☐ Grown using natural pest and weed control- better for the environment
- ☐ Contain more vitamins, antioxidants, and phytonutrients according to recent studies

Meat and dairy: Best (Grass fed/Pastured)

- ☐ Must be raised under specific animal welfare guidelines
- ☐ Cannot be given antibiotics or growth hormones, even when sick
- ☐ Must be provided with access to the outdoors
- ☐ Must be fed with 100 percent organic feed
- ☐ Cannot be fed animal byproducts or genetically modified (GMO) crops
- ☐ Must be fed feed produced on land that has been free from the use of toxic and persistent chemical pesticides and fertilizers for a minimum of three years
- ☐ Humane way to raise animals
- ☐ Better for the environment

Eggs: (Free Range/Pastured)

☐ Must come from farms that meet the USDA's national organic standards and are routinely inspected for compliance.

☐ Hens must be fed organic feed.

☐ Hens may not receive any antibiotics or hormones

☐ Must be allowed access to the outdoors and considered in a cage-free environment

☐ Humane way to raise animals

Organic labels:

☐ Farms must undergo USDA inspection and certification to bear the organic seal.

☐ Handlers and processors that work with the food before it reaches the market must be government certified as well.

☐ Meat marketed as "organic" must be 100 percent organic.

☐ Multi-ingredient products marketed with the USDA organic seal must contain 95 percent or more certified organic content.

Understanding Organic Food Labels, Benefits, and Claims

Organic food has become very popular. But, navigating the maze of organic food labels, benefits, and claims can be confusing. Is organic food really healthier? Is it more nutritious? What do all the labels mean? Why is it so expensive? This guide can help you make better choices about which organic foods are healthier for you, better for the environment, and how you can afford to incorporate more organic food into your diet.

Making a commitment to healthy eating is a great start towards a healthier life, and helps you take a load off so you can breathe better. Beyond eating more fruits, vegetables, whole gluten free grains, and good fats, however, there is the question of food safety, nutrition, and sustainability. How foods are grown or raised can impact both your health and the environment. This brings up the questions: What is the difference between organic foods and conventionally-grown foods? Is "organic" always best? What about locally- grown foods?

What are Genetically Modified Organisms (GMOs)?

Genetically Modified Organisms (GMOs) are plants or animals whose DNA has been altered. These products have undergone only short-term testing to determine their effects on humans and the environment.

In most countries, organic products do not contain GMOs.

The Benefits of Organic Food

Organic foods provide a variety of benefits. Some studies show that organic foods have more beneficial nutrients, such as antioxidants, than their conventionally-grown counterparts. In addition, people with allergies to foods, chemicals, or preservatives often find their symptoms lessen or go away when they eat only organic foods.

Organic produce contains fewer pesticides. Pesticides are chemicals, such as fungicides, herbicides, and insecticides. These chemicals are widely used in conventional agriculture and residues remain on (and in) the food we eat.

Why Do Pesticides Matter?

Children and fetuses are most vulnerable to pesticide exposure due to their less-developed immune systems, and because their bodies and brains are still developing. Exposure at an early age can cause developmental delays, behavioral disorders, respiratory issues, and motor dysfunction.

Pregnant women are more vulnerable due to the added stress pesticides put on their already taxed organs. Plus, pesticides can be passed from mother to child in the womb, as well as through breast milk. Some exposures can cause delayed effects on the nervous system, even years after the initial exposure.

Most of us have an **accumulated build-up** of pesticide exposure in our bodies due to numerous years of exposure. This chemical "body burden," as it is medically known, could lead to health issues such as headaches, birth defects, and added strain on weakened immune systems.

Organic food is often fresher. Fresh food tastes better. Organic food is usually fresher when eaten because it doesn't contain preservatives that make it last longer. Organic produce is often (but not always, so watch where it is from) produced on smaller farms near where it is sold.

Organic farming is better for the environment. Organic farming practices reduce pollution (air, water, soil), conserve water, reduce soil erosion, increase soil fertility, and use less energy. In addition, organic farming is better for birds and small animals, as chemical pesticides can make it harder for creatures to reproduce, and can even kill them. Farming without pesticides is also better for the people who harvest our food.

Organically-raised animals are not given antibiotics, growth hormones, or fed animal byproducts. The use of antibiotics in conventional meat production helps create antibiotic-resistant strains of bacteria. This means that when someone gets sick from these strains, they will be less responsive to antibiotic treatment. Not feeding animal by-products to other animals reduces the risk of mad cow disease (BSE). In addition, the animals are given more space to move around and access to the outdoors, both of which help to keep the animals healthy. The more crowded the conditions, the more likely an animal is to get sick.

Organic Farming and Locally-Grown Produce

Organic farming refers to the agricultural production systems that are used to produce food and fiber. Organic farmers don't use synthetic pesticides or fertilizers. Instead, they rely on biological diversity in the field to naturally reduce habitat for pest organisms. Organic farmers also purposefully maintain and replenish the fertility of the soil. All kinds of agricultural products are produced organically, including produce, grains, meat, dairy, eggs, fibers, such as cotton, flowers, and processed food products.

Essential characteristics of organic systems include:

☐ Design and implementation of an "organic system plan" that describes the practices used in producing crops and livestock products.

☐ Detailed record-keeping systems that track all products from the field to point of sale.

☐ Maintenance of buffer zones to prevent inadvertent contamination by synthetic farm chemicals from adjacent conventional fields.

Organic vs. Non-organic Produce	
Organic Produce:	Conventionally-Grown Produce:
No pesticides	*Pesticides used*
☐ Grown with natural fertilizers (manure, compost).	☐ Grown with synthetic or chemical fertilizers.
☐ Weeds are controlled naturally (crop rotation, hand weeding, mulching, and tilling).	☐ Weeds are controlled with chemical herbicides.
☐ Insects are controlled using natural methods (birds, good insects, traps).	☐ Insecticides are used to manage pests and disease.

Locally-Grown Fruits and Vegetables

What is local food? Unlike organic standards, there is no specific definition. Generally, local food means food that was grown close to home. This could be in your own garden, your local community, your state, your region, or your country. During large portions of the year, it is usually possible to find food grown very close to home at places such as a farmer's market. I enjoy getting to know my local farmers and supporting the ones who do their best to provide the best quality organic food.

There are great financial benefits when you buy locally. Money stays within the community and strengthens the local economy. More money goes directly to the farmer instead of to things like marketing and distribution.

Also, when you buy local, you are helping keep our air clean. In the U.S., for example, the average distance a meal travels from the farm to the dinner plate is over 1,500 miles. This uses a lot of fossil fuels and emits carbon dioxide into the air and causes more breathing issues. In addition, produce must be picked while still unripe and then gassed to "ripen" it after transport. Or the food is highly processed in factories using preservatives, irradiation, and other means to keep it stable for transport and sale.

Local food is the freshest food you can purchase. Fruits and vegetables are harvested when they are ripe and thus full of flavor and very yummy!

If you want garden fresh but don't have a green thumb or time to invest, consider a CSA (Community Supported Agriculture). The "bang for your buck" is incredible, and you get to try new veggies and fruits every time your order comes in!

Small local farmers often use organic methods but sometimes cannot afford to become certified organic. Visit a farmer's market and talk with the farmers around you. Find out how they produce the fruits and vegetables they sell. You can even ask for a farm tour, which I have done before with my kids. They loved seeing the gardens and petting the animals.

Fruits and vegetables where the organic label matters most	
According to the Environmental Working Group, a non-profit organization that analyzes the results of government pesticide testing in the U.S., the following 12 fruits and vegetables have the highest pesticide levels on average. Because of their high pesticide levels when conventionally grown, it is best to buy these organic.	
☐ Apples	☐ Kale
☐ Bell peppers	☐ Lettuce
☐ Carrots	☐ Nectarines
☐ Celery	☐ Peaches
☐ Cherries	☐ Pears
☐ Grapes (imported)	☐ Strawberries

Non-organic fruits and vegetables with low pesticide levels	
These conventionally grown fruits and vegetables were found to have the lowest levels of pesticides. Most of these have thicker skin or peel, which naturally protects them better from pests, and also means their production does not require the use of as many pesticides.	
☐ Asparagus	☐ Onion
☐ Avocado	☐ Papaya
☐ Broccoli	☐ Pineapple
☐ Cabbage	☐ Peas (sweet)
☐ Corn (sweet)	☐ Sweet potatoes
☐ Eggplant	☐ Tomatoes
☐ Kiwi	☐ Watermelon
☐ Mango	

Does Washing and Peeling Get Rid of Pesticides?

Rinsing reduces, but does not eliminate, pesticides. Peeling some-times helps, but valuable nutrients often go down the drain with the skin. The best approach: eat a varied diet, wash all produce, and buy organic when possible.

One way to help is to make a veggie/fruit wash with lemon essen-tial oil. I fill my kitchen sink with water and add 5 drops of my lemon oil and soak them for 20—30 minutes. You can also use 1/2 white vinegar. Sometimes I combine the two. The lemon oil removes the wax and toxins and also keeps the produce fresh.

Organic Meat and Dairy

Organic meat, dairy products, and eggs are produced from animals that are fed organic feed and allowed access to the outdoors. They must be kept in living conditions that accommodate the natural behavior of the animals. Ruminants must have access to pasture. Organic livestock and poultry may not be given antibiotics, hor-mones, or medications in the absence of illness; however, they may be vaccinated against disease. Parasiticide (a substance or agent used to destroy parasites) use is strictly regulated. Livestock dis-eases and parasites are controlled primarily through preventative measures such as rotational grazing, balanced diet, sanitary hous-ing, and stress reduction.

Organic vs. Conventional Meat and Dairy	
Regulations governing meat and dairy farming vary from country to country. In the U.S., these conventionally-raised meats and dairy products were found to have the lowest levels of pesticides.	
☐ Organic meat and dairy: ☐ No antibiotics, hormones, or pesticides are given to animals ☐ Livestock are given all organic feed. ☐ Disease is prevented with natural methods such as clean housing, rotational grazing, and a healthy diet. ☐ Livestock must have access to the outdoors.	☐ Conventionally-raised meat and dairy: ☐ Typically given antibiotics, hormones and feed grown with pesticides ☐ Livestock are given growth hormones for faster growth. ☐ Antibiotics and medications are used to prevent livestock disease. ☐ Livestock may or may not have access to the outdoors.

Organic food buying tips

Buy in season – Fruits and vegetables are cheapest and freshest when they are in season. You can also find out when produce is delivered to your market. That way, you know you're buying the freshest food possible.

Shop around – Compare the price of organic items at the grocery store, the farmer's market, and any other venue (even the freezer aisle!). Purchase the most economical ones. If local is not available, we shop at Costco and Trader Joe's. These two stores are the most reasonable in price when you are buying organic in bulk. Having three kids means buying food all the time, so I am so thankful my husband works at Costco because I am always telling him to bring this and that home.

Remember that organic doesn't always equal healthy – Junk food can just as easily be made using organic ingredients. Making junk food sound healthy is a common marketing ploy in the food industry, but organic baked goods, desserts, and snacks are usually still very high in sugar, salt, fat, or calories.

Chapter 12

ANSWERS TO DIABETES

Davaid age 37 was living with type 1 diabetes for 6.5 years, and he never understood why, but was always curious to figure it out.

He wanted to get a handle on his diabetes and understand more about his autoimmune disease. He wanted to find out what was going on with his thyroid numbers. He wanted answers.

After coming to one of Dr. Weaver's wellness seminars, he knew this was the place he should go. He found great support to live a healthy lifestyle through meeting with Dr. Weaver. The focus on his disease was always to get to the root of the problem, so that that the problem can be dealt with.

He learned that what he ate was so important to his healing. He ate OK before, but now he is making much healthier choices.

At first, eliminating gluten, dairy, and soy was tough, but later, he found out it wasn't necessary in his diet and other foods taste better. Getting to really know his body and what foods he needed to avoid was interesting and very helpful. In order for his diabetes to be better, he had to first renew his mind, which led to permanent results.

So many people like David go through life not knowing what the true cause of their dis-ease is. David was very eager to learn, and I was able to teach him why his body was in that dis-ease pattern. Again, my goal is get your body to be at its optimal and so you can fulfill your God-given purpose.

David's wife was his big support in his healing. She was the one to help him with his meal planning and preparation.

Food plays a role in many aspects of our life, from celebration to sorrow. The last thing you want is a long-term rigid list of rules about what to eat. Good nutrition is more than just rules. No matter the basis of your personal food decisions, finding a balance and peace with food is key to a lifetime of health and well-being.

Information-based decisions are the most important aspects of a healthy diet. It involves making choices that allow flexibility, and doesn't just follow rigid dietary rules. In fact, strict dietary rules often lead to failure in the long run—and it's the long run that you must always be thinking about with your dietary regimen. If you can't see yourself on a program for the rest of your life, you are looking at the wrong program. Yes, the program must evolve as new information becomes available to you, but you are moving from a life-long program that works for you to a life-long program that works even better. My information-based program gives you plenty of flexibility in your long term choices.

I love teaching the fundamental principles of self-care with information. It has pulled so many of my patients from the brink of despair. But once you know the principles, you are the one who must employ them to embrace your wellness lifestyle. Even your level of self-education will evolve. These simple guidelines will get you started:

Forego Processed Foods – Minimize or avoid foods that come out of a box, a wrapper, or as a bottled drink other than water (of course, there are exceptions to the box-wrapper-bottle avoidance).

☐ Forgo baked goods (cakes, brownies, rolls, biscuits,), cereal (Wheaties, Cap'n Crunch, Raisin Bran), pasta (macaroni and cheese), prepared sweets (cookies, candy bars, cinnamon crackers), sodas, juices, and other sweetened drinks.

- ☐ Perimeter Shop – The perimeter of the grocery store is filled with both the healthiest and the freshest food. Avoiding the center aisles will save you from unhealthy food, and just may save you money.
- ☐ Eat Raw – Provides higher levels of nutrition, essential digestive enzymes and cofactors, and have less chance of food reactivity. In addition, this helps you eliminate or reduce your consumption of processed foods.
- ☐ More Vegetables – You need the enzymes in fruits and vegetables.
- ☐ Supplementation – You may be missing key vitamins and minerals.
- ☐ Less Cooking – Overcooking can destroy essential nutrients.
- ☐ Eliminate Sugar – Sugar in all its many forms stresses the body.
- ☐ Eat at Home – There's nothing as genuine, good as a home-cooked meal, especially when your husband cooks it.

Chapter 13

NO MORE DEPRESSION

In Jessica's words, *"God led me to Dr. Weaver in October of 2004 at a volunteer event when I was 22 years old and at the lowest point in my life. At that time, I was struggling with many health issues, including severe acid reflux, depression, anxiety and irritable bowel syndrome. I had been struggling with these for over 5 years (since my junior year in high school). My parents had taken me to numerous doctors and specialists, ranging from my pediatrician to Duke Hospital to a regular chiropractor. Nothing had helped, not even the surgery for acid reflux, which was the last effort. I was truly at the end of my road after spending my high school and college years at numerous doctor appointments and given multiple tests every time school was out. I was suicidal and just wanted the Lord to take me from this Earth. I started receiving upper cervical care from Dr. Weaver. Within 18 months, I was prescription free due to chiropractic care and supplements. Thankfully, I haven't been on any prescriptions since for any of the health issues I was dealing with. It was a true miracle for me to no longer have any symptoms of acid reflux, depression, anxiety, or irritable bowel syndrome. Dr. Weaver was able to pinpoint my issue immediately, and I never had any neck/back pain through the years. All my problems started in February 1999 after a wreck I was involved in. I had x-rays at the time of the wreck, and of course, the ER physician said everything was fine...just had whiplash and it would be better in about 2 weeks. Just take the prescription pain pills. My soreness was gone, but all the other health issues I mentioned previously began within a month.*

Fast forward 12 years later…I still receive upper cervical care every 3 weeks as do my husband, two sons, grandparents, and mother. Dr. Weaver was one of my biggest supporters through pregnancy. I didn't have any issues at any point in time. My 13-year-old son no longer has any asthma symptoms since receiving upper cervical care, and hasn't had a sick visit with pediatrician in 4 years. My youngest son started chiropractic care immediately, within 12 hours of being born, he had his first upper cervical correction. He is now 3 years old and has never had a sick visit with the pediatrician. He has only been for preventative visits. He takes supplements daily, and he loves the essential oils Dr. Weaver recommends. At the first sign of any sickness, we start the essential oils, load up on supplements, and run to Dr. Weaver's office for upper cervical chiropractic care, and 99% of the time we need to be adjusted, and are back on par within a day or two.

I am extremely thankful God lead me to Dr. Weaver 12 years ago. I feel 100% that if he had not, I would not be where I am today, and possibly not even on this earth still striving to serve Him. Thank you Dr. Weaver for your wonderful care and allowing my body to heal itself naturally without drugs. Your love, care, and commitment to my family is amazing, and we are all forever grateful. I have no idea what we would do without you and upper cervical care. You are truly a Godsend. You are my "life line." Much love to you and may God continue to use you to bring healing to people's lives. Look forward to many more years."

This last testimony I couldn't leave out. It was hard to pick a handful, but I wanted to pick the most valuable ones that went with my book. As tears stream down my face, I am here to tell you I am just a plain ol' country girl that God is using to help bring healing to others. All I wanted to do was to help one person, and today, I have helped thousands regain their health. I give all the glory to God because He was the one who created my healing hands and opened up my heart to care for others. I hope these stories speak to your heart and help you see the LIGHT!!

Now you know why I say I can trace every ailment we face today to improper breathing. If I teach you nothing else from this book, my website, and our e-mail messages, it is that "For BREATH is life, and if you BREATHE well, you will live long on earth."-Sanskrit Proverb

God BLESS and I love you all.

—*Dr. Corinne Weaver, DC*

REFERENCES

1. Arbes, S. J.Jr., Gergen, P.J.et al. Prevalences of positive skin test responses to 10 common allergens in the US population:results from the third National Health and Nutrition

2. America Faces Allergy/Asthma Crisis. www.acaaiorg.2007

3. Rios,J.L. and Recio, M.C. Medicinal plants and antimicrobial activity. *J Ethnopharmaco. 2005;100(1-2):84.*

4. Li T,Peng T. Traditional Chinese herbal medicine as a source of molecules with antiviral activity. *Antiviral Res.* 2013 Jan;97(1):1-9.

5. Reichling J, Schnitzler P, Suschke U, Saller R. Essential oils of aromatic plants with antibacterial, antifungal, antiviral, and cytotoxic properties—an overview. *Borsch Complemented.* 2009 Apr;16(2):79-90.

6. Carson, C.F.; Hammer , K.A.; and Riley, T.V. Melaleuca alternifolia (Tea Tree) oil: a review of antimicrobial and other medicinal properties. *Colin Microbial Rev.* 2006;19(1):50-62.

7. Chattopadhyay I, Biswas K et al. Turneric and curcumin: Biological actions and medicinal applications. Current Science 2004;87(1):44-53

8. Bryer E. A literature review of the effectiveness of ginger in alleviating mild-to-moderate nausea and vomiting of pregnancy. J Midwifery Womens Health, 2005; 50(1):e1-3.

9. Grzanna R, Lindmark L, Frondoza CG. Ginger-an herbal medicinal product with broad anti-inflammatory actions. J Med Food. 2005;8(2):125-32.

10. Braun JM, Schneder B, Beuth HJ. Therapeutic use efficiency and safety of the proteolytc pineaople enzyme Bromelain-POS in children with acute sinusitis in Germany. In Vivo. 2005 Mar-Apr;19(2):417-21.

11. Buttner L, Achilles N, Bohm M, Shah-Hosseini K, Mosges R. Efficacy and tolerability of bromelain in patients with chronic rhinosinusitis-a pilot study. B-ENT. 2013;9(3):217-25.

12. Goncagul G, Ayaz E. Antimicrobial effect of garlic (allium sativum). Recent Pat Antinfect Drug Discov. 2010 Jan;5(1):91-3.

13. Inoue T, et al. J Cardiol. 2008. Tropical fruit camu-camu (Myrciaria dubia) has anti-oxidative and anti-inflammatory proberties.

14. Paul J, Gnanam R, Jayadeepa RM, Arul L. Anti cancer activity on Graviola, an exciting medicinal plant extract vs various cancer cell lines and a detailed computational study on its potent anti-cancerous leads.

15. Frieri M, Valluri A. Vitamin D deficiency as a risk factor for allergic disorders and immune mechanisms. Allergy Asthma Proc. 2011 Nov-Dec;32(6):438-44

16. Peat, J.K., Mihrshahi, S.et al. Three-year outcomes of dietary fatty acid modification and house dust mite reduction in the Childhood Asthma Prevention Study. J Allergy Clin Immunol. 2004; 114 (4):807-813.

17. Jirillo E, Jirillo F, Magrone T. Healthy effects exerted by prebiotics, probiotics, and symbiotic with special reference to their impact on the immune system. Int J Vitam Nutr Res. 2012 Jun;82(3):200-8

18. Boyle, R. J. and Tang, M.L. The role of probiotics in the management of allergic disease. Colin Exp Allergy. 2006;36(5):568-576

19. Fraker, P.J.; King, L.E. et al. The dynamic link between the integrity of the immune system and zinc status. J Nutr. 2000;130 (5S Suppl):1399S-1406S.

20. Thormar, H.; Isaacs, C. E.; Brown, H. R.; Barshatzky, M. R.; Pessolano, T. (1987-01-01). "Inactivation of enveloped viruses and killing of cells by fatty acids and monoglycerides". Antimicrobial Agents and Chemotherapy. 31 (1): 27–31. doi:10.1128/aac.31.1.27. ISSN 0066-4804. PMC 174645. PMID 3032090.

21. Arora, Rajesh; Chawla, R.; Marwah, Rohit; Arora, P.; Sharma, R. K.; Kaushik, Vinod; Goel, R.; Kaur, A.; Silambarasan, M. (2011-01-01). "Potential of Complementary and Alternative Medicine in Preventive Management of Novel H1N1 Flu (Swine Flu) Pandemic: Thwarting Potential Di-

sasters in the Bud". Evidence-Based Complementary and Alternative Medicine. 2011: 1–16. doi:10.1155/2011/586506. ISSN 1741-427X. PMC 2957173. PMID 20976081.

22. Litonjua, A.A. Rifas-Shimar, S. L. et al. Maternal antioxidant intake in pregnancy and wheezing illnesses in children at 2 y of age. Am J Clin Nutr. 2006; 84(4):903-911.

23. Middleton E Jr, Drzewiecki, G., and Krishnarao, D. Quercetin: an inhibitor of antigen-induced human basophil histamine release. J Immunol. 1981; 127(2):546-550.

24. Martinez-Losa, M. J.et al nhibitory effects of N-actylcysteine on the functional responses of human eosinophils in vitro. Colin Esp Allergy. 2007;37(5):714-722.

25. Wuyts, W. A., Vanaudenaerde, B.M. et al. N-acylcysteine reduces chemokine release via inhibition of p38 MAPK in human airway smooth muscle cells. Euro Repair J. 2003; 22(1):43-49.

ABOUT THE AUTHOR

D r. Corinne Weaver, DC, has been a lifelong resident of North Carolina. She received her pre-chiropractic educational requirements at the University of North Carolina at Wilmington. She earned her Bachelor of Science degree in Biology and Chemistry from Excelsior College. Dr. Weaver attended Life University School of Chiropractic, where she graduated Cum Laude with her Doctor of Chiropractic degree.

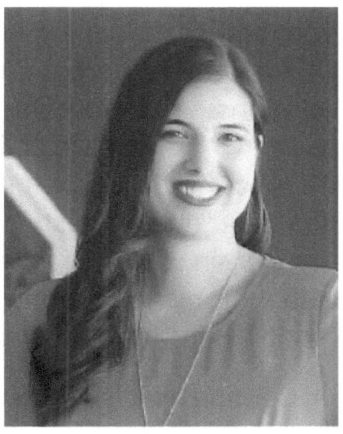

During her childhood, Dr. Weaver had issues with asthma and allergies that she thought she would always have to endure. After her first upper cervical adjustment at age 21, her health began to improve with upper cervical care and natural herbal remedies. This brought about a drug-free wellness lifestyle for her and her family, and she enthusiastically discovered her calling of helping others heal naturally.

Since 2004, Dr. Weaver has been the clinic director at Upper Cervical Wellness Center, a complete health and wellness center that promotes holistic healing and improved quality of life. Upper Cervical Wellness Center is known for finding the root cause of health concerns through lifestyle changes, diagnostic testing, nutraceutical supplementation, and correction of subluxation—as opposed to medicating the symptoms. The practice offers cutting-edge technological care at its state-of-the-art facility, including laser-aligned Upper Cervical X-rays, bioimpedance analysis (measuring body composition), digital thermography (locating thermal abnormalities characterized by skin inflammation), and complete nutritional blood analysis, which is focused on disease prevention.

Education is a key to success for Dr. Weaver's clients. The curriculum includes nutrition, simple cooking techniques, detoxification, organic shopping on a budget, fitness, exercise, stress management, and herbal-o-logy (natural herbs and home remedy solutions). With its commitment to having a personal and caring relationship with each client, the practice successfully helps people who are experiencing symptoms, such as pain and inflammation; migraines; digestive issues; ear infections in infants and children; brain dysfunction; asthma and allergies; unexplained weight gain; chronic fatigue; high blood pressure; depression and other mood disorders; blood sugar imbalances; and sleep problems.

Dr. Corinne Weaver, DC, was recently named one of Charlotte Magazine's "Top Doctors" for 2016 and is now #1 international bestselling author.

Contact Information

Dr. Corinne E. Weaver, DC

14015-D East Independence Blvd.

Indian Trail, NC 28079

Websites:

www.drcorinneweaver.com   www.getwellnc.com